The IV Solution

AF113080

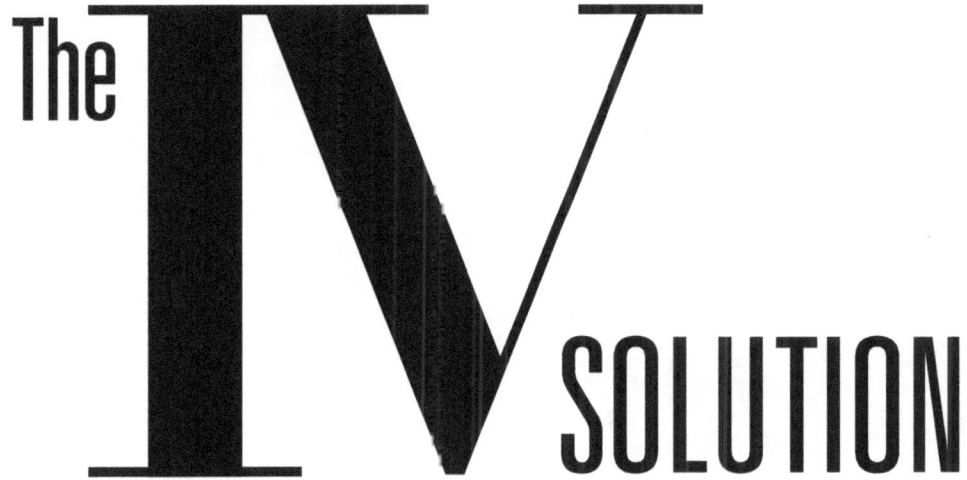

Reclaim your wellness with **micronutrients**

Dr. Tara Campbell, BAH, ND

© 2023 Tara Campbell, BAH, ND

Published by Conversation Publishing.
www.conversationpublishing.com

All rights reserved. No part of this book may be reproduced or used in any manner without the prior written permission of the copyright owner, except for the use of brief quotations in a book review.

To request permissions, contact the author.

Printed in the United States of America.
First paperback edition August 2023.

Cover and layout design by G Sharp Design, LLC.
www.gsharpmajor.com

ISBN 979-8-9852879-8-1 (paperback)
ISBN 979-8-9852879-4-3 (ebook)

To every single patient I've met. You have helped me grow both professionally and personally. I'm grateful for the opportunity to share in your individual journey of health. Thank you.

To my family, friends, mentors, teachers, and colleagues — all those who have championed me along the way as I hope to have championed you.

To my G and G, whose hearts are smiling here and above.

To my parents, whom have always encouraged and supported me in every endeavor, dream, and goal.

To Jay, my partner in life, love, and business. Thank you for believing in me beyond what I thought possible. There's momentum in the right now! (Just remember who has the needle!) I love you.

And to our daughter, Ellie, who lights the way and whom we do it all for.

TABLE OF CONTENTS

Preface: Our Post-Pandemic Wellness Opportunity ix

PART I 1
Reclaim Your Wellness with Micronutrients

Chapter 1 Getting to the Root of Our Wellness Problem 3
Chapter 2 Back to Basics: What Our Body Needs 33
Chapter 3 The IV Solution 55
Chapter 4 What's Your Vision of Wellness? 75
Chapter 5 Your Blueprint for Higher Health 87

PART II 107
Your How-To Guide to IV & Micronutrient Wellness

How IV Vitamin Therapy Can Help You... 109
1. Improve Low Energy 111
2. Support Digestion (Gut Health) 113
3. Care for Your Vision 117
4. Support Your Immune System 119
5. Promote Weight Loss and Benefit Metabolism 123
6. Support Surgery Recovery 127
7. Reduce Menstrual Cramping 129
8. Alleviate Allergies and Asthma 133
9. Support Brain Health 135
10. Address Brain Fog 137

11. Improve Degenerative Disc Disease
    and Chronic Pain.................................... 141
12. Support Postpartum Depression 145
13. Enhance Skin Health................................. 149
14. Support Fertility and PCOS 153
15. Alleviate Migraines and Concussion Issues........... 157
16. Get Better Quality Sleep 161
17. Support Fibromyalgia 163
18. Improve Cardiovascular Health..................... 165
19. Enhance Physical Performance 169
20. Support Opti-Aging................................. 171
A Closing Word on Your Wellness 175

PREFACE:
OUR POST-PANDEMIC
WELLNESS OPPORTUNITY

As I wrote this book throughout 2020 and 2021, I had more people than ever visit my clinic to talk about their health. Being a naturopathic doctor, I've spent my whole career talking about health and wellness. But suddenly, my patients weren't just curious—there was an urgency to their health questions.

> *How can I feel good again?*
> *Where do I start? Do I need a lifestyle 180?*
> *What am I doing right now to impede my health and how do I stop?*
> *What would happen if I don't make any changes?*
> *What if I'm doing everything "right," but still don't feel great—what then?*

The pandemic showed many of us that our wellness is a top priority. If we eat better, we feel better. If we're active and mobile, we feel stronger. If we give our bodies the nutrients we need, we can add years to our lives.

With this renewed attention to our wellness, we have the opportunity to be healthier and feel better than ever before.

Wellness, at its most basic level, means your body performs optimally. You can use energy and recharge. You can be exposed to wear and tear on your muscles or body through everyday living, and still have the resilience and ability to repair your body naturally. Wellness is when your body is recharging, replenishing, and restoring on its own. But for most of us, our body needs help. To achieve optimal performance, we must embrace these three aspects of our wellness: mindset, movement, and micronutrients.

We are most familiar with the first two. We know we must have a wellness mindset, develop habits, and have positive reinforcement—with consistency—to remain healthy. We also know the power of movement in keeping us in good physical and mental shape.

But most of us are unfamiliar with the role of micronutrients. *Aren't these just food?* Not quite.

Micronutrients are the vitamins and minerals your body needs to perform optimally. Vitamin C, vitamin D, B vitamins, magnesium, calcium, selenium, zinc, and more. Food delivers these vitamins, minerals, and amino acids through the digestive system before they get into the bloodstream, where they are absorbed by our cells and then delivered to wherever the body needs them. But for many of us, no matter how healthy we try to be, we remain micronutrient deficient—and it's getting worse. Today, more and more studies reveal North Americans to be chronically deficient in the basic nutrients we need to maintain our health.[1,2]

For much of my early life, I likewise struggled with micronutrient deficiency—and I didn't even know it. As a teenager, I pushed

---

1 JoAnn E Manson et al., "Vitamin D Deficiency – Is There Really a Pandemic?," *The New England Journal of Medicine* 375, no. 19 ((November 10, 2016): 1817-20, https://doi.org/10.1056/NEJMp1608005.

2 Opinder Sahota, "Understanding Vitamin D Deficiency," *Age and Ageing* 43, no. 5 (2014): 589-91, https://www.ncbi.nlm.nih.gov/pmc/articles/PMC4143492/pdf/afu104.pdf.

myself, both in school and as a long-distance runner, but I kept hitting a wall. I was easily run down, and struggled with significant periods of anxiety and depression. I reached a point of complete burnout, finally needing medical attention. I was disheartened by the only recommendation: take a pharmaceutical medication. If it didn't work, I was told I would need to try another medication.

I earnestly asked my doctor, "Isn't there a test we can do to see what's going on with me?" I sensed there had to be something more to it that wasn't being addressed. I was terrified to put a pharmaceutical into my body that was going to alter my brain chemistry without clearly knowing what was causing the problem.

I spent a long time looking for an approach that resonated with me—an approach that made sense. I finally discovered evidenced-based naturopathic medicine. Naturopathic doctors seek to understand the whole of your health—how all body systems work together, because when one system is affected, it has a ripple effect throughout the whole body.

Naturopathic doctors make it a top priority to *care* for your complete wellness rather than treat individual symptoms or "dis-ease" in isolation. You are a whole person and must be treated as a whole. The goal is empowering your wellness—bringing your body and mind back into alignment and balance.

Finally! I thought. I felt enormous relief. This discovery has been life-changing for me and countless others like me. The experience was so powerful that I vowed to make a career of it. At naturopathic school to become a naturopathic doctor (ND), I learned the science behind the health issues I experienced in my early years as well as a holistic understanding of how issues develop overtime. Ever since, it's been my goal to share this wellness-based approach with as many people as possible.

When you are deficient in nutrients such as vitamin C, magnesium, vitamin D, and antioxidants, there's a negative ripple effect throughout your entire body. Your energy doesn't fully recharge when depleted. Any bump or injury, however minor, doesn't fully heal, causing inflammation, oxidative stress, and further nutrient depletion.

From low energy to brain fog, mood concerns to sleep difficulties, and stubborn weight loss to vulnerable immune systems, there are dozens of wellness struggles that I see at my clinic every day that have a root cause in micronutrient deficiency.

But there's hope!

While conventional medicine treats sickness and disease, it is evidence-based naturopathic medicine that works to optimize your overall wellness. Why not give your body the nutrients it needs to heal itself before it turns into something that needs medical attention?

I've dedicated my practice to my patients' overall wellness. A big part of our team's work is replenishing micronutrients with IV therapy. The IV bag—a solution often comprised of saline or sterile water and vitamins like C, B, minerals, and amino acids—delivers micronutrients directly into your bloodstream, bypassing the digestive system, so that your body can most effectively receive the nutrients it needs to refresh, restore, and revitalize.

IV nutrient therapy is a relatively new health phenomenon, but its clinical use has been around for decades. While it's grown in popularity over the past few years to become one of the most in-demand wellness treatments, many of my patients have questions about their wellness related to micronutrient deficiencies, and the role that IV therapy can play.

That's why I wrote *The IV Solution*—to share with you how we have come to this place of micronutrient deficiency, what conditions it causes, and what you can do about it to reclaim your wellness.

PART I
Reclaim Your Wellness with Micronutrients

"Your body works hard to absorb what you put in it, so give it the best."

NORMA KAMALI[3]

"Nutrients are not drugs and they can't be studied as drugs. They are part of a biological system where all nutrients work as a team to support your biochemical processes."

DR. MARK HYMAN[4]

"Silent epidemics of vitamin and mineral deficiencies [are] affecting people of all genders and ages."

THEODORE H. TULCHINSKY, MD, MPH[5]

---

3 Norma Kamali, *Norma Kamali: I Am Invincible* (New York: Abrams, 2021).

4 Mark Hyman, "Why You Should Not Stop Taking Your Vitamins," *Dr. Hyman* (blog), website for Dr. Mark Hyman, "Why You Should Not Stop Taking Your Vitamins," the "Articles" page, the website for Dr. Hyman, October 18, 2011, https://drhyman.com/blog/2011/10/18/why-you-should-not-stop-taking-your-vitamins/

5 Theodore H. Tulchinsky, "Micronutrient Deficiency Conditions: Global Health Issues," *Public Health Reviews* 32 (2010): 243-55, https://doi.org/10.1007/BF03391600.

CHAPTER 1

GETTING TO THE ROOT OF OUR WELLNESS PROBLEM

Melissa thought she would never run again. A mother of four teenagers, she had been highly active with them and supported her children in their competitive sports. She took pride in being able to keep up, especially since she'd just turned fifty. She thought that as long as she was healthy, she could keep up with her athletic family.

Then she hurt her back. At first, it would only flare up whenever she'd been active. But as the months went by, it lingered more and more, until it was a constant acute pain. Maybe the pain would disappear?

After another month of pain, Melissa was talking one day with her good friend Sabrina, who happened to be a patient of mine. She winced as they talked, the back pain now chronic, and burst into tears.

"I'm healthy and active," Melissa lamented, "so what's going on with my body?"

Sabrina had been going to our clinic to improve her overall wellness after struggling for years with dragging energy, a low immune system, and sleep concerns. She knew there might be a connection between Melissa's overall health and her body's ability to function pain-free, and that IV therapy could be beneficial.

Acting on Sabrina's recommendation, Melissa visited our clinic. As her naturopathic doctor, I listened to her story. At this point, even though Melissa hadn't been running for three months, the pain would still flare up doing normal activities around the house. "Oh mom, not again!" her kids would say whenever she keeled over in pain after trying to do simple tasks like tying her shoes.

"Will it just get worse with age?" she asked me.

On top of the back pain, Melissa was suffering periodic anxiety and occasional migraines, which she'd had for decades and considered normal at this point. But I knew there was more to the story.

Melissa reminds me of the many patients I see at our clinic. Every day, people walk in with questions and concerns about their health. They have symptoms like back pain, anxiety, low energy, lack of sleep, migraines, inflammation, hypertension, and more. For these issues, they've seen medical doctors, who might offer medication without any further attention to important lifestyle aspects like nutrition, exercise, and mindset.

Everyone wants to do better for their health. Some don't know where to start. Others believe they are doing the best they can, but it's simply not enough. *What then?*

As Melissa shared her story, I could tell she was frustrated. She'd treated her back pain with massage and chiropractic care, and had been tested with CT scans and an MRI to see if she needed surgery—which her doctors told her she didn't. Their recommendation: "Reduce exercising when it gets too painful and take an over-the-counter anti-inflammatory medication."

It's a hopeless feeling to do your best and still end up struggling. "I'm not the me I usually am," she said to me, clearly at a low point.

Thankfully, there was a lot we could do to help Melissa. My hunch was that her body was revealing the most common health issue I see: *nutrient deficiency*. In other words, her body either wasn't getting or wasn't absorbing the nutrients it needed for optimal function, causing warning signs such as the back pain flare ups as well as anxiety.

> Her body was revealing the most common health issue I see: *nutrient deficiency.*

Even though she ate healthy food, took vitamin supplements, and was in great shape, she was still micronutrient deficient. No matter how fit we are or how well we think we "take care" of ourselves, if we're not getting enough of the right nutrients delivered to our cells, then various symptoms will show up.

At our clinic, Higher Health Naturopathic Centre and IV Lounge, we treat many patients with intravenous vitamin therapy. This treatment delivers micronutrients (vitamins and minerals) directly into the patient's bloodstream where nutrients are absorbed in order to improve overall cellular function. When our cells are working better, our whole body works better. Our wellness improves, and many symptoms can disappear when cells have the vitamins and minerals they need to function optimally.

Studies have shown most people in North America are chronically deficient in magnesium, vitamin D, and B3.[6] Even a minor magnesium deficiency "may lead to changes in gastrointestinal, cardiovascular, and neuromuscular function. Physical exercise may deplete magnesium, which, together with a marginal dietary magnesium intake, may impair energy metabolism efficiency and the capacity for physical work."[7] Vitamin D deficiency, meanwhile, "is associated with muscle weakness," in addition to mood changes, cardiovascular health, a weakened immune system, and more.[8]

When it comes to our immune system, researchers publishing in the US National Institute of Health (NIH) note, "Adequate intakes of vitamins and trace elements are required for the immune system to function efficiently. Micronutrient deficiency suppresses immune functions ... and leads to dysregulation of the balanced host response. This increases the susceptibility to infections, with increased morbidity and mortality."[9]

The volume of research begs the question: *Why are so many of us micronutrient deficient?*

The greatest contributor to this deficiency is our modern lifestyle and all the activity, stress, and dietary factors that play into it. And, despite our best efforts, micronutrient deficiency tends to worsen with age. As we get older, "diet alone may be insufficient and tailored

---

6 A.A.A. Ismail, Y. Ismail, and A.A. Ismail, "Chronic Magnesium Deficiency and Human Disease; Time for a Reappraisal?" *QJM: An International Journal of Medicine* 111, no. 11 (November 2018): 759-63, https://doi.org/10.1093/qjmed/hcx186.

7 Caroline H. Bohl and Stella L. Volpe, "Magnesium and Exercise," *Critical Reviews in Food Science and Nutrition* 42, no. 6 (2002): 533-63, https://doi.org/10.1080/20024091054247.

8 Opinder Sahota, "Understanding Vitamin D Deficiency," *Age and Ageing* 43, no. 5 (2014): 589-91, https://www.ncbi.nlm.nih.gov/pmc/articles/PMC4143492/pdf/afu104.pdf.

9 Eva S. Wintergerst, Silvia Maggini, and Dietrich H. Hornig, "Contribution of Selected Vitamins and Trace Elements to Immune Function," *Annals of Nutrition and Metabolism* 51, no. 4 (2007) 301-23, https://doi.org/10.1159/000107673.

micronutrient supplementation based on specific age-related needs [are] necessary."[10]

In treating Melissa, we started with our normal foundation, which is an IV once per week for four weeks to introduce the body to the basic micronutrients we need at a higher level than can be obtained through food alone: vitamin C, B vitamins, magnesium, calcium, minerals, amino acids, antioxidant support (NAC, glutathione), and vitamin D. Our cells and in particular the mitochondria, need these micronutrients to stay humming. Hydration from the IV solution is also key.

By her third session, Melissa walked in glowing. "I know this isn't a placebo," she said excitedly, "because my back is feeling so much better. I even went for a run the other day, and it didn't hurt! And my massage therapist said my back feels different," likely because of improvements in tissue quality.

After her foundational series, Melissa continued with treatment at our clinic, receiving a weekly IV for eight weeks, and then a monthly IV thereafter. Getting rid of her back pain helped reduce her anxiety, and her migraines became far more infrequent.

In continuing to receive IV nutrient therapy, she was no longer merely treating her pain. She now had a new perspective on her overall wellness. "I feel more vibrant, more alive, more energized. I have changed my overall perspective of wellness. I am excited about health and empowering my body." When combined with other healthy lifestyle measures, like exercise and learning how to prepare healthier food at home, Melissa noted: "The IV treatment gave me back my life."

---

10 Silvia Maggini, Adeline Pierre, and Philip C. Calder, "Immune Function and Micronutrient Requirements Change Over the Life Course," *Nutrients* 10, no. 10 (2018): 1531, https://doi.org/10.3390/nu10101531.

Her wellness improved so much that she had bigger goals in mind.

A year after walking into our clinic with frustrating back pain that had sidelined her from running, Melissa competed in a marathon. She finished with little of the post-race pain she used to feel. At the finish-line, she wept, thankful she could stay mobile and active with age.

"At 55, I feel I am in better shape than most of us in our thirties, both physically and mentally. I wish I knew back then what I know now."

She's not alone. No matter how healthy we try to be, most of us remain micronutrient deficient—and it's getting worse. When you are deficient in nutrients such as vitamin C, B vitamins, magnesium, amino acids, vitamin D, and glutathione, you may experience a negative ripple effect of health symptoms throughout your entire body. It can feel like you're totally out of control of your health.

Thankfully, there's hope!

In order to reclaim our health, first we must get to the root of our wellness problem. We must look deeper than conventional medicine's "sickness" model, which treats symptoms, to arrive at the wellness model of naturopathic medicine, which sees the whole picture of our health—how our body works as a whole, harmoniously optimizing functions, repairing and replenishing, balancing hormones and neurotransmitters (like serotonin, GABA, and Dopamine), and bringing wellness treatments down to the cellular level. Most of all, we must understand the foundation of our wellness is cellular health, and that the IV is the most direct way to deliver the micronutrients our cells need.

I've dedicated my practice to helping my patients get to the root of their overall wellness and to replenishing micronutrients with IV therapy. In this book, I share with you both *why* we have come to this place of micronutrient deficiency and *how* IV therapy can help remedy common wellness issues we struggle with. Whether you read a specific chapter of interest or every page, this book will help you reclaim your wellness.

Our Wellness Problem

Do you feel in control of your wellness?

Whether or not you struggle with one or more health concerns—high blood pressure, sleep difficulties, anxiety, or others—there are times when we all feel our health is out of our control.

2020 was a year when many of us rediscovered the importance of our health. As a pandemic spread globally, claiming lives and changing our habits, many of us looked with newfound importance at our wellness. We started eating right, working out, taking supplements, and more. For some, though, this wasn't enough. And for others, it got even worse.

Melissa's story is representative of many of us and our health today. We have a health issue, but don't understand the underlying cause. So we treat the symptom, rather than addressing our body's needs. In doing so, we never feel entirely in control of our wellness. What's missing?

After working with thousands of patients, I've found wellness problems arise when we ignore our *cellular health*. To a great degree, our wellness is dependent on the health of our cells. If you're burning out, then likely your cells are burning out, too.

> If you're burning out, then likely your cells are burning out, too.

We are each made of trillions of cells. Like us, our cells regularly face health challenges. Cells get damaged, inflamed, old, tired, and weakened by toxins from our air, water, and food intake. For our cells to remain healthy, they constantly strive to repair, replenish, and detoxify—all of which require micronutrients.

Today, our modern lives contribute a great deal to our micronutrient deficiency. We live in a world of chronic stress. Whether it be finances, work, our environment, a global pandemic, or even the daily ups and downs of life, stressors are all around us.

Our wellness *problem* is simple to define: as our lifestyle weakens our cellular health, we don't do enough to provide the micronutrients our cells need to remain healthy. This wellness problem surfaces in various ways, with "symptoms" that make us wonder:

- *Why can't I lose weight?*
- *Are my hormones out of balance?*
- *Why can't I sleep?*
- *Why do I get colds and feel run down so often?*

To regain control of our wellness, we must focus on the underlying cause of these symptoms to find the root, which is often related to micronutrient deficiency.

15 Common Wellness Struggles (And How Each Relates to Micronutrient Deficiency)

In the past decade, I've worked with thousands of patients who have had a range of diverse issues. Despite the differences, one aspect of their health causes or exacerbates many of these issues: micronutrient deficiency. The good news: by providing more micronutrients to my patients, we've addressed their health issues and improved their overall wellness.

In speaking with patients, we always start by covering their concerns from head to toe. We go beyond the symptoms they're experiencing to understand what issues may be contributing to these symptoms.

Now, let's take a look at some common issues I hear from patients. *Do any of these struggles resonate with you?*

- Lack of sleep
- Low energy
- Inflammation
- Hormone imbalance
- Menopause/perimenopause, dysmenorrhea (painful periods)
- Stress
- Weight
- Immune (and autoimmune) concerns
- Digestive issues
- Environmental stressors
- Migraines and headaches
- Hypertension
- Neurodegenerative issues (such as Parkinson's, MS)
- Allergy/asthma
- Anxiety and depression

1. Lack of Sleep

I've treated many people who have a hard time falling asleep or who experience restless sleep. They say: "I'm waking every two hours and

I can't go back to sleep," or "I'm not dreaming anymore," or "I lie awake from 2 am to 5 am."

When they finally get out of bed in the morning, they feel terrible, and that feeling has become their normal. If this goes on for a long time, it can affect their life in numerous ways, with consequences such as brain fog, low productivity, weight gain, and feelings of sluggishness, agitation, and irritability.

Many overcompensate with coffee or other stimulants to keep going, then find those contribute further to their lack of sleep. It's a vicious cycle. Short-term solutions are often little better than a Band-Aid, doing nothing to actually remedy the issue. In fact, in the long-term, these "solutions" just make it worse.

The good news is that our sleep improves if we're providing our bodies the micronutrients we need. Patients notice they are less tired than before because of the nutrient replenishment.

When you're lacking micronutrients, your body isn't working as it should. Its function improves with micronutrient replenishment, which in turn improves sleep quality and vice versa. If you're not sleeping well, then you're not restoring your body or repairing cells, so they have to work harder to function, using more nutrients.

Research shows us the link between sleep and micronutrients: "Micronutrient status has also been linked to sleep duration, with sleep duration positively associated with iron, zinc, and magnesium levels, and negatively associated with copper, potassium, and vitamin B12 levels."[11]

---

11 Xiaopeng Ji, Michael A. Grandner, and Jianghong Liu, "The Relationship Between Micronutrient Status and Sleep Patterns: A Systematic Review," *Public Health Nutrition* 20, no. 4 (March 2017): 1-27, https://www.ncbi.nlm.nih.gov/pmc/articles/PMC5675071/pdf/nihms916373.pdf.

2. Low energy

I see many patients who say they struggle with low energy. They don't necessarily have chronic fatigue syndrome—they just describe themselves as always being sluggish, foggy, unsatisfied, and unmotivated.

Many wonder: *Is it diet-related? Is it a hormone imbalance?*

More often, we find a micronutrient deficiency. When we do blood work, we're looking at levels of B12, vitamin D, ferritin, and thyroid indicators. We also want to know about inflammation, blood sugar levels, cholesterol levels, and hormones.

Sluggishness or fatigue can be a sign your cells are coping with inflammation and oxidative stress. Low micronutrients like vitamin D, B12, and iron could be a sign that you need a boost of them for your cells to surmount the challenges related to low energy.

Low energy could be a sign of something as commonplace as depriving your mitochondria (the energy-production center of every cell) of the nutrients they need to function optimally. "Adequate nutrient levels are essential for mitochondrial function as several specific micronutrients play crucial roles in energy metabolism and ATP-production.".[12]

3. Inflammation

Inflammation is present at the root of many health conditions.

At a cellular level, an injured cell can cause inflammation all around the cell. The redness of a knee injury, for example, is a sign the area is swarming with white blood cell-related particles in the bloodstream. With more particles crowding your blood, your cells have less access to micronutrients.

---

12 E. Wesselink et al. "Feeding Mitochondria: Potential Role of Nutritional Components to Improve Critical Illness Convalescence," *Clinical Nutrition* 38, no. 3 (June 2019): 982-95, https://doi.org/10.1016/j.clnu.2018.08.032.

It's like oil for a car: if you don't replenish your oil, it can get cruddy. The deteriorated oil can cause wear and tear, damaging the car's engine. It's the same with the crowding of inflammation. Oil in this example refers to the nutrients your body needs to replenish its circulation.

If you're eating nutrient-void food, like lots of sugar, then you're depriving your body of its ability to repair itself. This creates oxidative damage in the body—the sugar becomes an oxidant and causes inflammation. An issue with diabetes, for instance, is that there can be a lot of circulating sugar (glucose) in the bloodstream, causing, causing an oxidative process in your body that creates inflammation and can even lead to neurodegeneration.

There is a growing body of research into the phenomenon of inflammation. Researchers publishing in the NIH stated that, "an unresolved inflammatory response is likely to be involved from the early stages of disease development."[13] And, "Micronutrients contribute to the body's natural defences on three levels by supporting physical barriers (skin/mucosa), cellular immunity and antibody production."[14] These are just some examples of how micronutrient deficiency pairs with inflammation.

4. Hormone imbalance

We often see patients with hormone concerns. With aging and every day stress comes a change in hormones. You make less, which can have a ripple effect throughout the body.

---

13 Anne M. Minihane et al., "Low-grade Inflammation, Diet Composition and Health: Current Research Evidence and Its Translation," *British Journal of Nutrition* 114, no. 7 (October 2015): 999-1012, https://www.ncbi.nlm.nih.gov/pmc/articles/PMC4579563/pdf/S0007114515002093a.pdf.

14 Silvia Maggini et al., "Selected Vitamins and Trace Elements Support Immune Function by Strengthening Epithelial Barriers and Cellular and Humoral Immune Responses," Supplement, *British Journal of Nutrition* 98, no. S1 (Oct. 2007): S29-35, https://doi.org/10.1017/S0007114507832971.

Replenishing your cells with micronutrients is an anti-aging (opt-aging) approach. While we don't use the IV to directly balance hormones, vitamin therapy does improve cellular health, which in turn improves hormone production, vitality, and overall well-being.

We never just treat your "hormones" or your "thyroid." Instead, we get to your underlying wellness to improve the functions of your hormones and thyroid. Micronutrient deficiency, over time, can cause your body to manifest symptoms of dysfunction. Replenishing nutrient deficiencies could go a long way in correcting most all hormone imbalances, from thyroid to adrenal and inflammation to specific hormone conditions.

Then there's adrenal fatigue, which makes you feel like you're completely out of gas, as if everything is sluggish and not working. We often consider a hormone issue like adrenal fatigue as a mitochondrial issue, because the mitochondria need micronutrients to power your adrenal glands.

What fuels your mitochondria and cells are hydration and micronutrients, which in turn helps your adrenals to make hormones and glucocorticoids (think cortisol).. Conventional medicine may treat a hormone imbalance with prescription medication, while an IV with antioxidants, vitamins, minerals, and amino acids may improves underlying cellular health and metabolic flow, which in turns may help your body to function and respond more effectively..

5. Menopause/perimenopause, dysmenorrhea (painful periods), and PCOS

If you have painful periods due to menstrual cramping, then magnesium helps reduce cramping. I have many clients who come in before or during cramping for IV treatment and benefit from the magnesium.

Hormone imbalances can manifest at any age. For women in their thirties, we can see perimenopause-like symptoms from imbalances in estrogen, progesterone, DHEA, testosterone, and cortisol. For women in their forties and fifties, we often see a correlation between low B vitamins and low vitamin C in relation to estrogen and progesterone, suggesting a strong micronutrient deficiency over time.

To understand what your body needs, we look at your bloodwork. If specific hormones are high or low, there's often an origin related to micronutrient deficiency.

Why do some people sail through menopause while other people don't? In our experience, there are health markers related to wellness and micronutrient intake that show us how symptom-heavy the journey can be. Melissa, whose story opened this chapter, sailed through menopause. I'd like to think her reclaiming her wellness had a lot to do with it.

> ## Why do some people sail through menopause while other people don't?

For women with polycystic ovary syndrome (PCOS), research shows they "often have higher levels of inflammation and oxidative stress and lower levels of magnesium and glutathione. In fact, studies show that women with PCOS have almost 50 percent lower glutathione levels compared to controls."[15] Such research concluded that nutrient supplementation helped women manage their PCOS.

15 Elif Günalan, Aylin Yaba, and Bayram Yilmaz, "The Effect of Nutrient Supplementation in the Management of Polycystic Ovary Syndrome-Associated Metabolic Dysfunctions: A Critical Review," *Journal of the Turkish-German Gynecological Association* 19, no. 4 (December 2018): 220-232 https://www.ncbi.nlm.nih.gov/pmc/articles/PMC6250088/.

6. Stress

I see a lot of deficiency in B vitamins when it comes to clients reporting stress. For myself, I have a history of stress, anxiety, and depression. By doing blood work and genetic testing, I discovered I had a predisposition to B6 deficiency. After burning out on my B6 stores, I'd feel more stressed.

Science knows the relationship between B vitamins and stress. When you're stressed, you're using your B vitamin stores. By stocking up, we can lower our susceptibility to stress.

Most everyone nowadays is reporting they're stressed out. Our response is to have B vitamins in every IV we give. IV is more effective than taking B vitamins orally, as it can take a long time to see a response with oral intake. If someone is so depleted by their lifestyle and stress, they may not have any positive response to an oral B vitamin at all. At that point, true replenishment typically comes with IV.

7. Weight

So many patients ask, "Can you help me lose weight?" The answer is yes, most certainly—but not in the way you might expect.

Most people have been misled into thinking about weight loss in terms of restriction: fewer calories, smaller portions, avoiding specific foods, less fun.

But I think of it from a point of view of *super nutrition*. Managing your weight isn't about starving yourself for the sake of a caloric deficit—it's about remedying your sluggish cellular function. You may need to get *more* micronutrient intake than you're already getting. Hence, you might find it surprising that you need to eat *more* of some foods—a lot more.

Your toxicity over time, and wear and tear, can also kick your mitochondria to the floor, which impacts your weight and metabolism. To restimulate mitochondria and your metabolism, you may need a boost of micronutrients, which you often can't get from food alone, especially through a caloric deficit.

I've seen plenty of patients switch from a "deficit" mentality to an "abundance of the right things" mentality, getting the right nutrition, movement, and hydration, then enjoying the profound effect this switch has on their weight.

8. Immune concerns

A low immune system is a sign your body is not working well. You're not resilient; your body's resistance is down and you're more susceptible to attack. Why does your immune system weaken?

Typically, it's because your body lacks micronutrients. It's common knowledge that vitamin C is good for your immune system, but why (and at what dosage)? Basically, it's one of the main cellular nutrients in counteracting oxidants.[16] Zinc, too, plays a role, reducing oxidative stress and balancing the white blood cell (lymphocyte) response to injury.[17] Protein, and its amino acids, are likewise essential for your immune system—and these are also key ingredients in IV therapy.

For all immune concerns, there's an inflammatory aspect, with cells attacking other healthy cells. Researchers at the NIH have noted

---

16 Wintergerst, Maggini, and Hornig, "Contribution of Selected Vitamins," https://doi.org/10.1159/000107673.

17 Anuraj H. Shankar and Ananda S. Prasad, "Zinc and Immune Function: The Biological Basis of Altered Resistance to Infection," Supplement, *The American Journal of Clinical Nutrition* 68, no. 2 (August 1998): 447S-63S, https://doi.org/10.1093/ajcn/68.2.447S.

the connection between vitamin C, enhanced cortisol production, and the "clinical control of immune disorders."[18]

9. Digestive Issues

Many of us struggle with digestive issues, such as bloating, gas, constipation, diarrhea, and gastritis. Often, a major contributing factor to digestive issues is diet, inflammation, and compromised nutrient absorption.

Acidity, like inflammation, can create a breeding ground for disease. Inflammation is a leading cause of acidity, which disrupts our gut bacteria, predisposing us to imbalance. Healthy bacteria can't flourish in an acidic environment. Usually when there's acidity, it's caused by a poor diet and sugar, the presence of which over time causes chronic digestive inflammation, dysbiosis, and impaired nutrient absorption.

Alkalizing the body reduces inflammation, enhances nutrient absorption, and improves body functioning. Our blood is basic, or alkaline. A healthy diet and quality rest helps keep the body alkaline.

In IV therapy, when using vitamin C (which is typically acidic), we use ascorbate, a form of vitamin C that is more alkaline, and we pair it with bicarbonate, to further ensure the solution is similar to the blood's PH. Vitamin C helps repair the body so it can filter out acidic waste through our kidneys, liver, and lymphatics. This helps restore alkalinity in the body by clearing acidity. Improving digestive health further enhances micronutrient absorption.

---

18 M. Kodama et al., "Vitamin C Infusion Treatment Enhances Cortisol Production of the Adrenal via the Pituitary ACTH Route," *In Vivo* 8, no. 6 (November – December 1994): 1079-85, https://pubmed.ncbi.nlm.nih.gov/7772741/.

10. Environmental stressors

As many of us live in cities, there are environmental factors that are stressors on our health. The big one in urban areas is *oxidative stress.*

In *The End of Alzheimer's*, author Dr. Dale E Bredesen describes how inflammation, toxicity, and micronutrient deficiency are the three major causes of Alzheimer's.[19] In particular, oxidative stress manifests in aging, due to wear and tear on the system.

We're exposed to all kinds of oxidants (often called "free radicals") in our daily modern life. When you walk down the street, you're breathing in oxidants, which are unstable molecules trying to become stable by stealing electrons from other cells. The more electrons the invading oxidants take from our cells, the more damage and inflammation they cause to our cellular health. This causes our cells to restore and repair, along with a cascade of other responses in our body.[20]

If we're constantly immersed in oxidants, our cells linger in a chronic state of repair, with a desperate need for micronutrients and antioxidants. That's how oxidative stress can become a significant cause of micronutrient deficiency. Without the needed micronutrients, our body suffers a lot of wear and tear on the system. Alzheimer's is just one of many outcomes after years of oxidative stress.

That's why we take antioxidants through food and supplementation, to provide the extra electrons our cells need to quench oxidants and prevent the wear and tear. Bottom line: you repair better when your cells work better.

---

19 Dale E Bredesen, *The End of Alzheimer's: The First Program to Prevent and Reverse Cognitive Decline* (New York: Avery, 2017).

20 V. Lobo et al., "Free Radicals, Antioxidants and Functional Foods: Impact on Human Health," *Pharmacognosy Reviews* 4, no. 8 (July – December 2010): 118-26, https://doi.org/10.4103/0973-7847.70902..

For many of my patients, learning about oxidative stress and repairing cells is a light bulb moment. "I never thought about it that way, but I can totally see what's happening to me."

A few years ago, we had an event with Dr. Walter Crinnion, ND, a pioneer in environmental medicine who has sadly since passed. He explained how those who live within a mile of a major highway in a major population center likely have a high environmental toxic load. Toxins found in such things like automobile exhaust find their way into our body as oxidants. "Health studies show elevated risk for development of asthma and reduced lung function in children who live near major highways," among other concerns.[21]

These toxins clog your system, particularly your glutathione pathway, which antioxidants need to reach our cells. In such an environment of excess oxidative stress, your glutathione pathway can become sluggish and exhausted. The micronutrient that best helps your glutathione pathway continue functioning is magnesium, which we commonly use in IV nutrient therapy for this very reason, along with actual glutathione and NAC (a precursor to glutathione).

11. Migraines and headaches

We approach headaches with a similar investigation of a patient's underlying wellness. One patient, Terry, is a former hockey player who experienced several concussions. Years later, he still hadn't fully recovered, despite giving up the sport and doing his best to take care of his health. He regularly had migraines and brain fog, likely because the initial damage to his brain had yet to heal.

---

21 Doug Brugge, John L. Durant, and Christine Rioux, "Near-Highway Pollutants in Motor Vehicle Exhaust: A Review of Epidemiologic Evidence of Cardiac and Pulmonary Health Risks," *Environmental Health* 6 (August 2007): 23, https://doi.org/10.1186/1476-069X-6-23.

Our hunch was that he hadn't fully replenished his cellular health to support ongoing healing. In treatment, our goal was to further stimulate his body's ability to repair.

> **In treatment, our goal was to further stimulate his body's ability to repair.**

Concussions are a shock to the system. It's like crashing a car: you have to repair the car, not drive around in a wreck expecting it to function the same.

Once he began receiving IV nutrient therapy, his system received the nutrients needed to make repairs. Within a few short months, his brain fog cleared up and his migraines all but disappeared.

12. Hypertension

What is the root cause of high blood pressure? Is it inflammation-causing stress? Or magnesium deficiency? Liver health and congestion? Wear and tear on the heart, causing pressure to go up? There are several possible factors, each one requiring a different approach.

Getting to the root of hypertension allows us to find the right micronutrients to boost your health.

Research shows that micronutrients play a critical role in regulating blood pressure. Researchers at the NIH note the connection between minerals, blood pressure, and heart health: "Sodium, potassium, magnesium, zinc, selenium, copper, and calcium could directly or indirectly influence blood pressure."[22] While many take blood pressure medication to remedy hypertension, the same researchers note that "additionally, various anti-hypertensive drugs result in micronutrient imbalance, which ends up in poor vascular function and affects the overall health status."

13. Neurodegenerative Issues (Such as Parkinson's, MS)

When I see patients who have Parkinson's, MS, or other neurodegenerative issues, we explore oxidative stress, micronutrient deficiency, inflammation, and toxicity. "Oxidative stress, defined as the condition when the sum of free radicals in a cell exceeds the antioxidant capacity of the cell, contributes to the pathogenesis of Parkinson's disease."[23]

IV therapy provides an effective way to support your body's ability to manage the issue. In particular, glutathione, which repairs antioxidant function, can significantly reduce the severity of symptoms associated with Parkinson's. Glutathione directly "relates to protection of dopaminergic neurons from oxidative damage and its therapeutic potential in Parkinson's disease."[24]

14. Allergies/asthma

Did your doctor ever tell you that your allergies or asthma could be related to the micronutrients (or lackthereof) used by your cells? Probably not.

---

22 Hui-Fang Chiu et al., "Impact of Micronutrients on Hypertension: Evidence from Clinical Trials with a Special Focus on Meta-Analysis," *Nutrients* 13, no. 2 (February 2021): 588, https://doi.org/10.3390/nu13020588.

23 Michelle Smeyne and Richard Jay Smeyne "Glutathione Metabolism and Parkinson's Disease," *Free Radical Biology and Medicine* 62 (September 2013): 1-32, https://www.ncbi.nlm.nih.gov/pmc/articles/PMC3736736/pdf/nihms477670.pdf

24 Smeyne and Smeyne, 1.

Magnesium deficiency, in particular, has great implications for our allergies and asthma.[25] That's why magnesium sulfate is given in an IV in hospital settings to treat acute asthma.[26]

If you take an antihistamine to stop histamines, then vitamin C is essential. To get technical, vitamin C is anti-allergenic because it supports specific immune cells called mast cells. It's the stabilization of vitamin C to mast cells that prevents the release of histamines.

As researchers at the NIH confirm, "Vitamin C is important in mast cell activation disorder for its role in the breakdown of histamine and as a mast cell stabilizer."[27] When asthma inflames or obstructs your airways, additional key micronutrients such as copper, selenium, and zinc play a role in restoring respiratory functioning.[28]

15. Anxiety and depression

This struggle, for me, is personal. My interest in helping people achieve their best health started with my own health journey.

> **My interest in helping people achieve their best health started with my own health journey.**

---

[25] Jeroen H.F. de Baaij, Joost G.J. Hoenderop, and René J.M. Bindels, "Magnesium in Man: Implications for Health and Disease," *Physiological Reviews* 95, no. 1 (January 2015): 1-46, https://journals.physiology.org/doi/pdf/10.1152/physrev.00012.2014.

[26] Uwe Gröber, Joachim Schmidt, and Klaus Kisters, "Magnesium in Prevention and Therapy," *Nutrients* 7, no. 9 (September 2015): 8199-226, https://doi.org/10.3390/nu7095388.

[27] Alexandra R. Vaughn et al., "Micronutrients in Atopic Dermatitis: A Systematic Review," *The Journal of Alternative and Complementary Medicine* 25, no. 6 (June 2019): 567-77, https://doi.org/10.1089/acm.2018.0363.

[28] Dominika Zajac, "Mineral Micronutrients in Asthma," *Nutrients* 13, no. 11 (November 2021): 4001, https://doi.org/10.3390/nu13114001.

Growing up, I was an overachiever, trying to please everyone, and a marathoner—both literally and figuratively! I suffered periodic bouts of extreme anxiety, panic, and depression.

I didn't understand how I could feel so unlike myself at times. While I was healthy and active, I'd have many days where I felt truly disconnected from life, even though my logical side told me nothing was wrong. The truth was everything was wrong and being misperceived, and it was incredibly difficult to make it through the day.

One day, I went to my medical doctor. After a ten minute discussion, he handed me a prescription for an antidepressant medication. I remember that moment very clearly, because I was so shocked.

"Aren't you going to test me for anything?" I asked the doctor. "How do you even know this is the right medication for me?"

I was vulnerable and afraid, worried about how the medication would affect me. Mostly, I just wanted to understand the cause of my struggle.

The doctor simply answered, "There is no test. Take it for six weeks and then we'll check in. If you don't feel any different, we'll switch you to something else." Despite his good intentions, that only made me feel worse! Take a pill, and if it's wrong, take another?

I felt disempowered, disappointed, and disheartened. I was scared to put a chemical into my brain when they weren't sure it was right for me. *Wasn't there a better way to test what was going on with me? Wasn't there a better way to feel better?*

This experience started my journey of learning about the whole-systems approach to making sure the body is in balance. From there, I studied to become a naturopathic doctor.

In the course of my training, I came across a test that could show me my serotonin, dopamine, and adrenal cortisol levels—neurotransmitters and hormones that influence anxiety and depression.

One day, when I was feeling particularly low and not on any medication, I tested myself to see if I could figure out what was going on in my brain. My results showed very low serotonin, very low dopamine, and tanked adrenal cortisol.

To remedy these lows, I did a few things—botanical medicine for adrenal hormone balance, B vitamins and magnesium for cofactors to support neurotransmitter metabolism, and augmenting my serotonin and GABA with diet, exercise, and meditation. A short while later, when I was feeling better, I retested my levels. Sure enough, my neurotransmitters were balanced, but surprisingly, my adrenal production of cortisol was still low.

So, I took it on myself to support my adrenal glands and mitochondria. That's when I first started IV therapy, getting a weekly treatment of micronutrients. Not only would the IV give me all the above micronutrients, but it would give my adrenals the boost I otherwise couldn't get. Plus, the IV has the amino acid tryptophan, which provides cells with more building blocks to make serotonin. Conventional medicine may treat low serotonin with prescription medication, but an IV with more amino acids may have the same effect.

Treating my anxiety and depression from a cellular micronutrient-support standpoint seemed to be exactly what I needed. I felt great, but I wasn't certain of a connection until I tested myself again. I was floored by my results: I had normalized cortisol production from my adrenal glands to within a healthy range. The best part? My anxiety and depression were better than I could ever remember them being. While I can't claim this approach works for everyone, it did make me realize there was a strong connection between my anxiety and depression (neurotransmitter and hormone imbalances) and the micronutrients in my bloodstream.

Micronutrient Deficiency and Our Wellness

We are made of trillions of cells, all fighting for the same resources. Since they grab whatever they can from your bloodstream to repair, replenish, and detoxify, we need a constant supply of nutrients. Your cells are either sufficient or deficient in micronutrients, depending on how much is in your bloodstream. With fewer micronutrients, your cells don't work as well.

It's like a car: if you only put a quarter tank of gas in, it's not going to go as far as when your tank is full. We need to keep the tank full. The gas you're putting into your body is the nutrients that help it function: vitamin C, magnesium, calcium, vitamin D, amino acids, and more. These keep us going the distance.

The older we get, the more micronutrients we need in our bloodstream to function healthily. In other words, micronutrient deficiency contributes to the effects of aging. The older we get, the fewer vitamins we have. The more we need, the worse our cells are at replenishing and repairing.

In 2014, researchers published a study featuring experiments that used the blood of young and old mice.[29] The researchers put the blood of the old mice into the bloodstreams of the young mice, and the blood of the young mice into the bloodstreams of the old mice. The old mice with the young blood far outperformed the old mice

---

29 Dmytro Shytikov et al., "Aged Mice Repeatedly Injected with Plasma from Young Mice: A Survival Study," *BioResearch Open Access* 3, no. 5 (October 2014): 226-32: https://doi.org/10.1089/biores.2014.0043.

with old blood. The authors showed that nutrients in the bloodstream helped improve overall function.

Meanwhile, the young mice who received the old blood experienced decreased functioning, which means something more than their ability to filter blood was happening. The results showed that it was nutrients in the bloodstream that made functioning in the old mice cleaner and more nourishing.

The same goes for us humans. You have a better chance of recovering, repairing, and cleansing your functions with more necessary micronutrients in your bloodstream.

Look no further than those in our lives from older generations. Naturally, you see the signs of aging: wear and tear, thinning skin, blood vessel breakage, and more. It's no coincidence that an older person with blood vessel breakage is also vitamin C deficient. Blood vessels need vitamin C to remain elastic.

Vitamin C is an essential component of repairing blood vessels. When there's not enough of it, the vessels break down. As we age, and our vitamin C levels go down, we start to see more broken capillaries and blood vessels throughout the body.

Many of us are vitamin C deficient. We don't have scurvy, but as we age and experience different needs in our daily life, we end up using a lot of vitamin C. The only way we replenish it is through food like fruits, vegetables, and even meat. You may eat an orange and meet your required daily amount (RDA) of vitamin C, but is the RDA enough when every cell in your body uses it?

That's why it's so important to start taking care of the micronutrients in our bloodstream today. While it's not easy, my patients are always thrilled to learn that our cellular health is within our control. Cellular health depends on the basics of food, water, micronutrients, and light. We can thrive by getting back to these basics. The IV allows us to deliver the basic nutrients our cells need directly into our bloodstream.

If this approach sounds different than what you typically hear at your physician's office, then that's because it's based on the principles of evidence-based naturopathic medicine, which account for your whole-body health—putting you in control of your wellness.

The Naturopathic Approach to Addressing Our Wellness Problem

A medical doctor's job is primarily to *fix*. The medical doctor works within a system designed, above all else, to triage and treat symptoms and sickness.

Medical doctors trained in a specialty will treat a symptom or sickness depending on their specialty's training. That means the treatment occurs in isolation—your treatment begins and ends with the symptom or sickness.

Meanwhile, a naturopathic doctor's job is primarily to *care, support, and optimize*. The naturopathic doctor addresses your overall wellness. The benefit is that we look at your health through a wellness lens, helping you answer the question: *How can I feel my best?*

Conventional medicine may address symptoms of a viral or bacterial infection similarly for each patient—for example, with rest for viral infections, or antibiotics for bacterial infections.

Naturopathically, we are interested in understanding all contributing factors in catching a cold. We ask: *How often does the person get sick in a year?* If it's frequently, we would want to build up their immune resistance. We would also address any digestive health concerns, which often correspond with a cold or flu, as well as adrenal health, which corresponds to stress, sleep, hormone balance, and more. Nutrition (including micronutrient status) and lifestyle are likewise key in any naturopathic consultation, even if you "just have a cold."

The American Association of Naturopathic Physicians notes, "Naturopathic doctors are educated and trained in accredited naturopathic medical colleges. They diagnose, prevent, and treat acute and chronic illness to restore and establish optimal health by supporting the person's inherent self-healing process. Rather than just suppressing symptoms, naturopathic doctors work to identify underlying causes of illness, and develop personalized treatment plans to address them."[30]

The good news is we don't have to pick one or the other. Naturopathic medicine and conventional medicine are complementary, not mutually exclusive. They are both primary care providers. They both rely on the same science, research, and evidence-based foundation to medicine. The advantage comes not from choosing one or the other, but from having *both* options to support our wellness.

What I like best about being a naturopathic physician is that I get to really connect with my patients, taking the time needed to understand all aspects of their wellness—their main health concerns, past experiences, and overall life goals, as applied to their health.

An initial consultation lasts approximately 90 minutes, and forms the foundation of our work together. It is a health discovery session where we fully investigate all aspects of someone's health and lifestyle, as well as their complete medical and family history. It's important to investigate and understand all health concerns how they relate to and effect each other, rather than just looking at them in isolation.

---

30 "What is a Naturopathic Doctor?," The American Association of Naturopathic Physicians, accessed September 30, 2022, https://naturopathic.org/page/WhatisaNaturopathicDoctor.

For many patients, such sessions are the most amount of time they've ever spent thinking about or talking about their health with anyone, let alone a doctor.

This Book: Reclaim Your Wellness with Micronutrients

I believe that looking at our health with the wellness model rather than the "symptoms and sickness" model is the only way for us to truly *feel better*. In this way, we see micronutrients as essential for us to reclaim our wellness.

After founding my clinic, Higher Health, in 2014, and helping thousands of patients over the years, today we understand the power of looking at the roots of your wellness. We see the IV as one of several science-based solutions that help us deliver micronutrients to our cells, where they are needed most. These solutions also include several basics such as sleep, light, air, hydration, and diet, which I describe in the next chapter.

> My hope is that this book serves as your guide to reclaiming your wellness.

My hope is that this book serves as your guide to reclaiming your wellness. To that end, I've organized the book into two parts.

- In *Part I*, we explore the basics of our wellness and what we can do to reclaim it.
- In *Part II: Your How-To Guide to IV & Micronutrient Wellness*, we look at specific health struggles. Want to support your immune system? Lose weight? Combat allergies? Here you'll

find the common struggles alongside stories and practices of success.

Our goal for this book is that by the end, you say what Melissa told me excitedly on a recent visit: "I feel like 'me' again!"

CHAPTER 2

BACK TO BASICS: WHAT OUR BODY NEEDS

Christine was sick and tired of being sick and tired. A vice president of sales at a medical device manufacturing company, Christine traveled regularly. In those pre-pandemic days, Christine would say she spent half her life on an airplane. While she loved her work, the downside was its effect on her health.

"I would get three to four colds a year. They would last for a few weeks and would never seem to let up. This had gone on for years." The typical remedies—rest, fluids, vitamin C—were not enough.

Fed up, Christine decided to do something about it. After a recommendation from a friend, Christine came in for an appointment at our clinic, received her first IV treatment, and got blood work for continued customized IV therapy. She appreciated it when I told her, "When getting a series of IVs, it helps to have them customized for your body's needs."

Turns out, Christine's body needed a few essentials. Tests showed Christine to be low in B12, folate, B5, omega 3 fatty acids, vitamin D3, zinc, CoQ10, and vitamin C, while also being significantly sensitive to a host of foods (because of what's called a "heightened

IgG response," suggesting an exaggerated stress and inflammatory response in the body). And with her low immune health (overactive immune response IgG-wise), we recommended botanical-based immune builders, an anti-inflammatory diet personalized to taste and food preferences aligned with food sensitivity results, and a series of IV nutrient treatments (once a week for four weeks).

"The first few IVs, I had noticed I had more energy, but I was skeptical it might be a placebo effect," said Christine. "But as my regular monthly IVs progressed, I found myself getting stronger, with more energy than ever—and the best part about it was no flu or cold symptoms at all. It was as if my immunities had strengthened and could fight off most anything. Even when others were getting sick around me, I wasn't getting sick.

> **It was as if my immunities had strengthened and could fight off most anything. Even when others were getting sick around me, I wasn't getting sick.**

"My main condition was weak immune health due to stress at work and living a lifestyle where there's no time in the day to do anything related to self-nourishment for higher health. From travelling so much, I also found more often than not that I would get sick on long-haul flights, which would put a damper on the trip. I found by getting an IV the day before I flew out, my immune system would be much stronger, and I felt great when I arrived at my destination. The IV therapy pre- and post-travel provided me with confidence."

Additionally, Christine needed to address stress management with micronutrient replenishment. She is a fast-paced woman on the go, burning a lot of nutrient reserves to maintain function, while also being somewhat comfortable running on fumes (it takes one to know one!). Christine could manage, but at what cost? She was depleting her capacity to respond to stress, and health concerns were starting to present themselves. While some people may start to show a susceptibility to immune concerns, others may first reveal anxiety, mood, digestive, or sleep concerns. Overall, the underlying root cause is nutrient deficiency and wear and tear on the body.

With a bloodstream replenished with B12 and B vitamins in particular (our stress fighters!) and vitamin C, zinc, and magnesium, among others, Christine's cells had more resiliency to further moderate her immune response.

Three years later, at the time of this writing in 2022, Christine still hasn't been sick with another significant cold or flu. Both micronutrients and an understanding of Christine's immune system through bloodwork made a huge difference for her wellness.

It's not complicated. Our body needs a handful of basics to sustain its wellness. It's up to us to make sure we give our body the basics it needs.

Back to Basics

The number one conversation I have with patients is about getting back to the basics of our body and its rhythms. Our modern culture has become very good at teaching us how to go against our natural body rhythms. We burn the candle at both ends, spend too much time indoors, and don't sleep right. In doing so, our body learns *not* to trust us. We need to re-establish trust within our bodies to reclaim our health. We don't need a complicated diet or exercise regimen. Instead, we need to understand that our wellness is a lifestyle. A wellness lifestyle requires a few basics:

1. Sleep rhythms
2. Light exposure
3. Oxygen rich air
4. Hydration
5. Micronutrients/comprehensive nutrition

Throughout the book I describe mindset, movement, and micronutrient needs that contribute to a wellness lifestyle.

Here I describe the five basics, which primarily do one thing—support your cellular health. Getting back to basics is about getting down to the cellular level. It's about providing *more than* the minimum nutrients your cells need to survive, but enough so that they can thrive. With all the advances in our modern world and demands in our modern life, we simply *need* a higher quality of nutrition in order to keep up and minimize wear and tear.

THE MIGHTY MITOCHONDRIA

In particular, supporting cellular health means targeting the mitochondria, which is the core energy center of every cell. We remember from grade school science class that mitochondria are the powerhouse of the cell. But what does the mitochondria need to function as the powerhouse? A whole lot of B vitamins, vitamin C, and magnesium—the basic micronutrients.

Mitochondria use such vitamins in order to make ATP, which is analogous to gas for your car. ATP is the energy driving force or fuel, functioning as the principal molecule for storing and transferring energy in cells and then beyond to your whole body.

Let's look at vitamin C. Every cell in your body uses vitamin C, particularly the mitochondria within every cell. If you're getting your vitamin C through only one orange every day, then at a minimum you won't have scurvy. But your trillions of mitochondria will have a micronutrient deficiency.

Vitamin C reduces oxidative stress and inflammation, which we all have. After it's absorbed, it provides nutrients directly to your cells, contributing to your antioxidant pathways, quenching oxidants, and helping with cellular repair and inflammation reduction.

Since mitochondria need vitamin C and other nutrients, we target the mitochondria in everything we recommend. Whether it's light, air, water, nutrition, or the IV, getting micronutrients to mitochondria is the goal.

I have a patient whose husband is going through end-stage renal failure. She's wondering what's best for his health. His body needs nutrients, and dialysis, but how can we support his body's normal function as it endures these challenges? By ensuring we get as many micronutrients as possible to his cells without compromising function.

> According to researchers from the NIH: "Mitochondrial dysfunction…was found in…blood of end-stage chronic kidney disease patients regardless of hemodialysis."[31] The research showed vitamin C's potential to combat inflammation and oxidative stress, benefiting mitochondria in patients with renal failure.
>
> Even in complex cases like renal failure, the health basics—like getting nutrients to mitochondria—are paramount. So, how do each of these five basics benefit the body?

1. Sleep and rhythm

What is the advantage of a natural rhythm? Aside from just consistent sleep, there are innumerable benefits.

Wellness stems from a proper night's sleep, when you refresh and restore your body. If you don't get restorative nighttime sleep, your body is less able to replenish, repair, and restore for the following day. Over time, this sets the stage for a host of symptoms and chronic health conditions. Sleep and body rhythm is paramount to wellness. A body's rhythm can also be off because of cortisol or other hormone production levels, which rely on sleep.

Circadian Rhythm Disorder is not really talked about, yet it affects so many. Is your sleep-wake cycle out of sync and negatively impacting your health? It's all too common and highly treatable.

In fact, I would say sleep is one of the most important health factors to address. Throughout the pandemic, during lockdowns,

---

31 Patrick Chaghouri et al., "Two Faces of Vitamin C in Hemodialysis Patients: Relation to Oxidative Stress and Inflammation," *Nutrients* 13, no. 3 (March 2021): 791, https://doi.org/10.3390/nu13030791.

so many clients reported not getting out of their house until the afternoon. This means they were not seeing true sunlight until the afternoon, after likely sitting in front of a blue light computer screen all morning. And the saddest part is that children are living this way, too. We have to honor our circadian rhythms.

If you want to feel your best, it's important to align your sleep-wake cycle to cues from the environment, such as sunrise and sunset, or light/dark. You can also enhance circadian rhythm through consistent meal times and physical fitness routines. Modern-day living can throw us off kilter, and off healthy, natural, and normal body rhythms. This 100 percent affects your health.

Help your body and mind *trust* you again simply by stepping into the light first thing in the morning. I am also a fan of red-light therapy for circadian rhythm support.

In short: wake with the sun, get outside, rest when the sun goes down, try red light therapy, and let's chat further about balancing your circadian rhythm.

> In short: wake with the sun, get outside, try red light therapy, and let's chat further about balancing your circadian rhythm.

A symptoms-based model response to lack of sleep would be to prescribe you an antidepressant or a sleeping pill, not really considering *why* you're tired or the positive steps you could take to increase your sleep or rest or to simply empower balance. People often know why they are tired and unable to sleep. They just don't know what to do about it or how to change their lifestyle.

The sickness- and symptom-based model is based more on only treating whatever symptom you're experiencing at the moment, whereas the wellness model takes a larger view, looking at all factors, piecing together the puzzle, and creating small steps to promote health for the long term.

A wellness model of sleep explores several factors contributing to unrest, as well as the steps needed to repair your body rhythms, so that you can wake refreshed in the morning. It considers reasons for why you are tired and sluggish, possibly because your cells don't have what they need to carry on your daily function. Perhaps you lack the nutrients needed for optimal function? When it comes to insomnia, often hormone and neurotransmitter imbalances combined with nutrient deficiencies are the root cause.

A wellness model would look at the various factors contributing to fatigue.

- *How is your sleep?*
- *What are you eating?*
- *What times of the day are you eating?*
- *How is your digestion?*
- *Are you absorbing nutrients and clearing wastes effectively?*
- *What does your day look like?*
- *What time do you go to bed?*
- *What time of day does your body first see true sunlight?*

If you wake up and basically sit at your computer from 8:00 am until 9:00 pm, you certainly should feel tired and sluggish. You are throwing your body completely off its natural and intended rhythm, and your body will find a way to tell you that!

Let's teach your body to trust *you* again—to trust natural rhythms, routine, and order, to restore how your cells are meant to function.

2. Light

Light, first thing in the morning, is a must for health! We are meant to be exposed to the full spectrum of light. We're meant to be outside. As our modern lifestyles keep us indoors, we're not getting the full spectrum we need—meaning all the color rays of light, from red to white to UV. The more time we spend in front of a computer screen, wearing our clothes, getting indoor light, the more our body craves real light. This deficiency of natural light throws off our natural rhythms. It can cause illness, like seasonal affective disorder, which happens when we don't get enough white sunlight.

We get a lot of blue light from our computer screen, our phones, and our TVs. Lesser known but equally important is red light. For many of us, red is the main spectrum we're missing.

How often do you watch the sunrise and sunset like our ancestors who lived more in rhythm with the environment? Maybe, if you're lucky, you catch a beautiful sunset once every two weeks. But most people aren't so lucky. Missing out on the light from sunrises and sunsets throws off our circadian rhythm.

Exposing our brain to light first thing in the morning helps us later by stimulating our natural melatonin production, which is going to help you sleep at night. So if you want to improve your sleep, it's not always about addressing your bedtime routine—it's about your whole routine from the moment you wake up.

As red light supports everything from our mood to the production of ATP fuel for our mitochondria, we provide red light therapy at our clinic. Getting red light is a basic that helps put our body back into its natural rhythm—an essential in supporting our overall wellness.

VITAMIN D

Sunlight can provide us vitamin D, a hormone with multiple benefits for the body, from immune to cardiovascular health, to bone and brain health. Many are surprised to learn that even though they may spend "a lot" of time out in the sun, they aren't getting enough vitamin D.

Our body often has more need for vitamin D than what we can synthesize from exposure to the sun or from eating animal products. Especially for vegans, it's important to take the right form of vitamin D.

Our modern lifestyle has taken us out of the sunlight. It's also contributed to more physical, mental, and environmental stress. Both lack of sunlight and increased stress necessitate higher amounts of vitamin D.

Starting in 2020 during the pandemic, I began to notice more fatigue and low immune resistance. We starting testing vitamin D more, as research shows those who are more deficient in vitamin D were more susceptible to viral infection. "Vitamin D modulates the systemic inflammatory response through interac-

> tion with immune system," while deficiency is "also associated with worse severity and higher mortality" [32]
>
> From our testing, I've been surprised to discover how many of us are vitamin D deficient. The normal range is 75-250 nmol/L, but most people squeak just above 75 nmol/L, and others are more clearly deficient at around 20-40 nmol/L. That's just too low for an optimal immune and health response!

3. Air

Air is air, right? Not so fast. Research shows how dirty our air can be if we live in or near a city.[33] We should be mindful of the air quality we breathe, as low-quality air affects our cellular health.[34]

Iron, for example, doesn't bind onto the cells unless there's enough oxygen in the body. A lot of people who are iron deficient likewise don't have enough tissue oxygenation, preventing the iron from binding onto a cell. Glutathione also enhances your tissue oxygenation, which likewise enhances iron absorption.[35]

Air toxicity can also deplete your nutrients. If you're not getting enough oxygen in general into your bloodstream, then your body

---

32 Fausto Petrelli et al., "Therapeutic and Prognostic Role of Vitamin D for COVID-19 Infection: A Systematic Review and Meta-Analysis of 43 Observational Studies," *The Journal of Steroid Biochemistry and Molecular Biology* 211 (July 2021): 105883, https://doi.org/10.1016/j.jsbmb.2021.105883.

33 I.S Mudway, F.J. Kelly, and S.T. Holgate, "Oxidative Stress in Air Pollution Research," *Free Radical Biology and Medicine* 151 (May 2020): 2-6, https://doi.org/10.1016/j.freeradbiomed.2020.04.031.

34 Ramesha Chandrappa and Umesh Chandra Kulshrestha, "Major Issues of Air Pollution," in *Sustainable Air Pollution Management: Theory and Practice* (New York: Springer, 2016), 1-48, https://doi.org/10.1007/978-3-319-21596-9_1.

35 Francesca Silvagno, Annamaria Vernone, and Gian Piero Pescarmona, "The Role of Glutathione in Protecting Against the Severe Inflammatory Response Triggered by COVID-19," *Antioxidants* 9, no. 7 (July 2020): 624, https://doi.org/10.3390/antiox9070624.

will take the nutrients it needs from elsewhere. This will sink your body's efficiency, making it more acidic and causing more inflammation.

A wellness model considers the causes of your lack of oxygen. Is it from pollution? Or the functions of your body that aren't working properly?

> **MOLD AND CHEMICALS IN YOUR AIR**
>
> We have a lot of stories about people who visit us with health issues that don't seem right. After recommending they get an enivronmental air quality assessment, they discover mold, high dust counts, high electromagnetic frequency levels, or other concerns relating to water purity. Then, as soon as the mold is removed, all their health conditions evaporate!
>
> Mold is serious stuff. A lingering cough is a telltale sign your air quality isn't great. You may have a microorganism issue, like mold, or a chemical issue—like your carpet or the finishings on hardwood floors. When you're breathing in toxins, your body has to deal with the unclean air. The toxins disrupt cellular pathways, killing cells faster, depleting nutrients, and triggering an immune response, like flared allergies—or worse.

4. Hydration

This is one of the areas where the benefits of IV therapy for people in the modern world are most obvious. Many people do *not* drink enough fluids and walk around in a constant state of dehydration without realizing it.

A dehydrated person is like a wilting plant, even if only slightly wilted. We should perk up. Proper hydration can enhance energy, mood, mobility, and even hormone health. It can also decrease annoying aches and pains. "Overall, there is a growing body of evidence supporting the importance of maintaining a normal state of hydration on various health aspects."[36]

When it comes to water, the big topic to discuss is *absorption*. How much is your body absorbing?

> When it comes to water, the big topic to discuss is *absorption*. How much is your body absorbing?

The more you do for your health, the better you're able to absorb nutrients, which includes hydration. For example, if I were to set you up with your first IV, your body *wouldn't* be ready to fully absorb the micronutrients. If you've had a nutrient-depleting lifestyle, like sitting in front of your computer ten hours a day drinking coffee, then your body will struggle to absorb. The IV would go right through your body, like running water over dry soil. It's important to "teach" your body how to absorb the nutrients. We do this with incremental dose increases and consistency. In doing so, the dry soil becomes more moist and more able to absorb the added water and nutrients.

Your body has to *learn* how to absorb. If you were to start drinking five more glasses of water than usual, the first couple of days you're going to be running to the bathroom a lot. The good news is that,

---

36 DeAnn Liska et al., "Narrative Review of Hydration and Selected Health Outcomes in the General Population," *Nutrients* 11, no. 1 (January 2019): 70 https://doi.org/10.3390/nu11010070.

over time, your body and cells will learn how to absorb. You'll become more hydrated. The same with IV nutrients and hydration.

Initially, everybody has a different rate of absorption, and there's no way to know what it is. But the more consistent you are with wellness practices, the more you will start to optimize absorption.

Lastly—it's so important to drink good, clean water. It's easy to drink coffee and dehydrate yourself (and deplete minerals, as coffee demineralizes). I love my coffee, but I also make sure I have a lot of water and replenish micronutrients!

5. Food and micronutrients

The same goes for food—food-based and IV-based nutrients. I want people to start choosing food that builds up their micronutrient profile. I want to inspire people to pursue micronutrient-rich eating on their own. While I don't have customized recommendations for you in this book, just knowing that certain foods are micronutrient-rich should help you in your choices.

When there's inflammation, there's less absorption. The more inflammation you have, the more likely you are to have a leaky gut. The health practices we discuss, like healthy eating, reduce inflammation and repair the gut lining..

How so? Well, if you lack the nutrients needed for your cells to do the functions they're meant to do, then inflammation can persist. This can happen when you have a micronutrient deficit, or when you're not absorbing as you should.

If you're not absorbing properly, then the IV is a great way to receive necessary nutrients because it bypasses your digestive system and delivers nutrients directly into your bloodstream.

When we talk about naturopathic medicine, it's typically about healing from the inside out. But when it's the IV coming into the body, you're actually healing the outside of the digestion inwards. You're healing cells that will respond better to the food you eat and the nutrients you take.

If you only take oral supplements, and you already have an absorption or digestion issue, then it's going to take a while to overcome that challenge and recoup. IV-based nutrients help prop you up to respond better, so you'll get there faster.

The bottom line? Each day, you must ensure you exceed your micronutrient needs, and that you are absorbing those nutrients.

The Sickness & Symptom Model vs. The Wellness & Lifestyle Model

Most of us are familiar with the "sickness and symptom model" of our health. When thinking in the context of the sickness- and symptom-based model, we ask things like, "What's the fastest way to lose weight?"

We look at our health this way because we want to see results quickly. Unfortunately, health isn't achieved in that manner. There's no real shortcut to it. Instead, you've got to make sure you're covering all your bases. The *more* you do for your health, the *faster* you're going to get to where you want to go.

That's why I'm a proponent of a wellness lifestyle, or the "wellness and lifestyle" model of health, which gets us to the point of truly enjoying health. In a wellness lifestyle, you're always doing *more* than the bare minimum for your health, which has the effect of providing you ever-greater wellness.

> # In a wellness lifestyle, you're always doing *more* than the bare minimum for your health.

To live a wellness lifestyle, consistency is key, as are taking small steps, committing to it over a period of time, and leaning on the right support—such as working with a naturopathic doctor who can provide you the accountability, insight, and motivation you need to actually achieve wellness.

The wellness and lifestyle approach, focused on cellular and nutritive health and stimulating the mitochondria, is really a 24/7 commitment, which I think is refreshing to a lot of people who are used to the sickness and symptom model of conventional medicine. There's something *odd* about caring for our health only when we are sick or have symptoms.

There's a quote that comes to mind: "We're more motivated to move away from pain than we are to move towards pleasure." It's human nature. But rather than teaching patients how to run from pain, my focus is more about helping them move toward pleasure, helping them get excited about their health, and helping them accumulate small changes in their day that, over time, will make a big difference. After all, slow and steady wins the race.

I want you to feel vibrant. I want you to have energy. I want you to thrive, to be mobile, active, fit, clear-minded, focused, energized, and loving life—*at any age*. We can accomplish these things. But our goal won't ever be "lose weight as quickly as possible."

ANOTHER EXAMPLE: "I HAVE A LOT OF MUSCLE STIFFNESS AND PAIN."

The sickness model would prescribe you an anti-inflammatory. The wellness model would look at the quality of your muscles and tissue health: Do they have enough hydration? Are they being pulled in different directions or getting so much attention that there's inflammation? How can we restore normal functioning?

With muscle tension, we also look at nutrient deficiency. I would look at oxidative stress and accumulated toxicity, which causes more wear and tear over time. I would look at your posture: Are you hunched over your computer or cell phone all day? What about your sleep posture when you're laying down? What's your hydration like? What lifestyle factors are contributing to micronutrient deficiency, inflammation, and toxicity? These and more inform our response to "muscle stiffness and pain."

Your wellness lifestyle is all about accumulating the right choices when it comes to the basics. It's about tracking how you're trending and building momentum. The more choices you make to support your wellness, the healthier you'll be.

> Your wellness lifestyle is all about accumulating the right choices when it comes to the basics.

Think about your wellness this way—when you face any choice, ask: "Does this help my body/mind/cells or not?" That's a simple choice. Whether you're staring at a donut or about to watch *just one more* episode on Netflix before getting to sleep, it should feel empowering to know you're in such control of your health, and that the choices you make can improve your cellular health, making you more likely to feel replenished and recharged.

If you're not replenishing your tank, you're not keeping up. Eventually, it catches up with you. That's when people come to my office—when it finally caught up with them.

By then they have sinusitis, or constipation, or they can't sleep well, or they're anxious. Their health has slowly declined to the point where serious symptoms start to crop up. They don't feel as good as they used to because they have become depleted over time. It's a slow decline when not living a wellness-based lifestyle—then, suddenly, symptoms seem to appear overnight.

People say, "But I do all the right things. I eat well, I sleep, I exercise." The question I have is—how is your lifestyle supporting your cellular health?

You may be eating broccoli with dinner, but are you really addressing your wellness? Or are you just sometimes making a healthier choice, checking off a box or two, but not enough?

Your lifestyle must gel with your basic needs: light, sleep, air, hydration, and nutrients. For many people, the most challenging basic is getting enough micronutrients into their bloodstream.

Your lifestyle must gel with your basic needs: light, sleep, air, hydration, and nutrients.

I have a client, Phil, who is in his late 50s. He has a bit of a gut, so when asked about his health goals, he gave a very common response: "I really want to lose my belly." He had been struggling with his weight and wellness for a while. This past Christmas, his family bought him a Peloton bike, which they hoped might be the key to helping him gain control of his health. When I heard that, I wondered, *Is the answer really just a Peloton bike? Burning more calories, or pumping more blood, or building up your muscle? What about when he's not on the bike? What are his habits then? How is he sabotaging his health?* It's not about an hour on the bike a day, it's all the in between time that matters.

Using your body this way often isn't enough to support your cellular health. In other words, exercise is only *part* of a wellness lifestyle—and perhaps not even the most essential basic.

With Phil, even more than slimming down, he craved vibrancy so he could keep up with his active family. I showed Phil how he could achieve vibrancy with the IV (micronutrient replenishment). After a handful of sessions, he was feeling great—good enough to *enjoy* working out.

Many get it backwards. They think, "I need to work out to feel great." Oftentimes, it can be the other way around. Once you start feeling great, you are motivated to work out. Take care of your lifestyle, and your wellness follows.

Phil found that IV nutrient therapy and a wellness approach gave him the vibrancy he needed to change his lifestyle.

We don't need to feel guilty about our health; wellness can be fun. We can feel enlivened to make the right choices. It starts with understanding the basics our body's needs, and living a lifestyle to match.

THE SIX WEEK HEALTH SPRINT

In January 2021 at Higher Health, we launched a six-week "Health Sprint"—a focused IV series with testing, personalized nutrition, red light therapy, one-on-one health coaching, group connection, and full micronutrient support. My team of naturopathic doctors, a holistic nutritionist, and I were side-by-side with each client for six weeks, helping them implement specific strategies on a consistent basis to generate clear improvements in their health. Consistent connection and support, along with fine-tuning throughout the process, led to results such as micronutrient repair, and to a much greater understanding of lifestyle wellness. Participants even had a red light to take home, which complemented everything we were working on and further enhanced results!

Putting the goal directly in their hands (with support and guidance) made the difference. Our participants felt on target for sustainable results.

A six-week health sprint isn't about being perfect. A lot of people would come in disappointed, saying, "I didn't take my supplements," thinking they needed to do "all or nothing." In order to be healthy, you don't have to eat perfectly for six weeks. Your wellness is about trending upward. It's about making decisions on the whole, while knowing you don't have to be perfect all the time. Allow space for true wellness to happen and space for feeling connected to and supported by a community.

By incorporating small action steps on a daily basis, you become well on your way toward hitting your goal. That's why a six-week health sprint can be so powerful, because we're focused on your wellness with small, daily steps. You're not *allowed* to self-sabotage.

Our goal is to develop lifestyle habits that will continue beyond the six-week sprint. The more you can address health as part of your daily lifestyle, the better you're going to feel.

CHAPTER 3

THE IV SOLUTION

Janet was on the third week of a lingering cold. A marketing professional in her early thirties, she was go-go-go, pushing herself to the breaking point. Like many her age, she had an invincibility mentality. That, paired with a high-stress time in her life, had left her rundown. Burning the candle at both ends, the body eventually catches up with you.

While Janet exercised daily, ate a balanced diet loaded with superfoods like broccoli, and enjoyed overall excellent health, she was mistaken to think her body could "just take care of itself."

You can only run on fumes for so long. Eventually, your body tells you when it's depleted. For Janet, that surfaced as low immune resilience.

Persistent coughing, wheezing, feeling worse at night—Janet couldn't kick it. After a while, she asked me, "What can I do to beat this cold? I can't afford to be sick!"

I was in my first year of naturopathic practice, having just completed my IV licensing. My first recommendation was for her to take a specific immune supplement. I was so new to vitamin therapy that I didn't recommend the IV at first. I had yet to discover my love of IV and, frankly, I was still a bit apprehensive about vein insertion.

The symptoms persisted for Janet, who then asked me, "Isn't there anything stronger?"

"Well, there is IV nutrient therapy," I said. "It's the strongest, and it might be the best." Janet was keen right away. The thought of IV micronutrients piqued her interest, sounding like just what she needed. Frustrated by the cold, she was also ready and willing to do whatever it took to get better. Even though she was apprehensive about needles, she later told me, "I felt that the discomfort of the needle was going to be worth the benefits I was going to get out of it."

She was right. A few hours after the IV, Janet noticed she was starting to feel better. With the cold clearing up over the next couple of days, the experience made her a lifelong IV advocate.

Looking back, it's now clear that Janet had been depleting her B vitamin stores to a degree that her body benefited tremendously from a kick of B vitamins for stress and resilience; vitamin C for immune, adrenal, and cellular function; and magnesium to calm her nervous system.

Over the past decade, Janet has been a regular at our clinic to maintain her optimal wellness, and has learned to appreciate how the nutrients work for her. When she is run down, she always thinks of IV therapy first. "I always feel better in some way after each IV treatment. A couple of hours later, I notice more energy and I feel clearer and lighter. I have a really great sleep the night following an IV, and for the next few days, I notice an uptick in energy and feeling refreshed."

What about the colds?

"Touch wood, but I used to get sick quite a bit up until I started doing IVs. I would get a sore throat two to three times a year, plus ear infections. I'd take two rounds of antibiotics for that. My daily work life would always leave me run down, depleted, and more susceptible to catching something.

"Since my first IV, it's almost been a decade, and I can count the number of colds I've had on one hand—and not one them came close to needing antibiotics. Do I attribute this turnaround in my health to *only* the IV? Probably not. But it probably has something to do with it. Now I'll do an IV every 2 to 4 weeks, just for maintenance."

> "It's almost been a decade, and I can count the number of colds I've had on one hand."

After experiencing this turnaround in her health, and watching the same for thousands of other clients at our clinic, Janet has seen how the IV can help kickstart a healthier life. "The IV," Janet said, "becomes a catalyst to do a lot of other good things for our health in general. Oftentimes, if you're spending all this time and money getting IVs, you start to think, 'Well, I should be maintaining my wellness in other ways, too.'"

To this day, while Janet does a regular IV to help maintain optimal health, she's still no friend of needles. "Even today, it's the same thing. I still don't like a needle going in. Yet most of the time I barely feel it. But I do it anyway, because I know the results." Janet now considers an IV (along with chiropractic care) anytime she feels a headache coming on or feels generally run-down, as well as for muscle tension after intense workouts.

IV is not a magic cure, but it is a huge part of wellness. It helped Janet respond better to workouts and chiropractic adjustments by hydrating her muscles and nourishing cells.

In this chapter, we answer the most frequently asked questions about the IV.

After treating thousands of patients, we've heard it all. Whether you're curious about the IV ingredients, afraid of needles, or wondering what to expect on your first visit, this chapter helps you get to know the IV—one of our most powerful tools in reclaiming your wellness.

The Origins of IV Vitamin Therapy

Most of us are familiar with the IV therapy commonly used in hospital settings, where an IV bag delivers medicine or nutrients into a patient's bloodstream.

In this case, it's referred to as "parenteral nutrition" or TPN. A person may need TPN because of a gastrointestinal (GI) disorder or other issue that severely limits the ability of their digestive tract. A person may not be able to swallow food, move the food through the digestive system, or absorb nutrients from the food—conditions common to those with Crohn's disease, cancer, short bowel syndrome, or ischemic bowel disease.

However, critically ill patients who cannot receive nutrition orally for more than four days are also candidates for TPN.

Naturopathic medicine posits that if total parenteral nutrition is good for someone who can't eat, then it can also be good for optimizing your health. It makes sense to think that with improved nutrition, by any means, you can feel better. In the 1960s, Dr. John Myers, a physician from Baltimore, Maryland, pioneered a treatment of vitamins and minerals delivered intravenously.[37] He noticed the patients he was giving microdoses of vitamins to were doing better than his other patients who weren't taking the IV solution. Later dubbed the "Myer's Cocktail," it included magnesium, calcium, B vitamins, and vitamin C.[38]

In the years since Dr. Myers, other micronutrients have been found to be effective in treatments. The IV has likewise been used to treat a range of illnesses

While little was known about the IV a few decades ago, today an ever-expanding body of research shows its application in a number of studies.

Recently, researchers looked at using vitamin C as part of treating patients with COVID-19. "Previous studies have shown that vitamin C inhibited replication of some viruses such as herpes simplex virus, Epstein Barr, poliovirus, and influenza. There is potential utility in the use of vitamin C in viral infections and possibly COVID-19."[39]

Other research shows that, "High dose intravenous vitamin C appears to be remarkably safe. Physicians should inquire about IV vitamin C use in patients with cancer, chronic, untreatable, or

---

37 Alan R. Gaby, "Intravenous Nutrient Therapy: The 'Myers' Cocktail,'" *Alternative Medicine Review: A Journal of Clinical Therapeutic* 7, no. 5 (October 2002): 389-403, https://pubmed.ncbi.nlm.nih.gov/12410623/.

38 Alan R. Gaby, "Intravenous Nutrient Therapy: The 'Myers' Cocktail,'" Northern Centre for Integrative Medicine, uploaded May 2014, https://nc-m.ca/wp-content/uploads/2014/05/Myers-Article.pdf.

39 Raul Hiedra et al., "The Use of IV Vitamin C for Patients with COVID-19: A Case Series," *Expert Review of Anti-infective Therapy* 18, no. 12 (2020): 1259-61, https://doi.org/10.1080/14787210.2020.1794819.

intractable conditions and be observant of unexpected harm, drug interactions, or benefit."[40]

In recent years, most new patients walk in with the understanding that they need way more nutrients than those they get from food. Social media has played a big part in increasing awareness of the IV and its wellness benefits, as celebrities and health-conscious influencers have helped accelerate the prevalence of IV therapies.

LET'S TALK SCIENCE

IV therapy directly provides your cells with the specific nutrients and cofactors they need for optimal function. What do these terms mean?

A cofactor is the inorganic component (vitamin or mineral) that is needed to start an enzyme reaction in your body. An enzyme reaction is just a chemical reaction in a cell that is started (catalyzed) by an enzyme and a cofactor. These chemical reactions have to happen for your cells to transform the substances you put in your body into nourishing material. Since these reactions need a cofactor to get started, the more cofactors you have in your bloodstream, the more these nourishing reactions can happen.[41]

The IV delivers these micronutrients and cofactors directly into the bloodstream via a drip consisting of

---

[40] Sebastian J. Padayatty et al., "Vitamin C: Intravenous Use by Complementary and Alternative Medicine Practitioners and Adverse Effects," *PLos One* 5, no. 7 (2010): e11414, https://doi.org/10.1371/journal.pone.0011414.

[41] Bruce N. Ames, "Prolonging Healthy Aging: Longevity Vitamins and Proteins," *Proceedings of the National Academy of Sicences of the United States* 115, no. 43 (October 2018): 10836-44, https://doi.org/10.1073/pnas.1809045115.

> the nutrients dissolved in a solution, which also serves to hydrate you. In addition to hydration, the IV benefits you because the bioavailability of the content is 100 percent—that is, the nutrients go directly into your bloodstream, rather than being partially filtered out by your digestive system or your liver. For that reason, the trillions of cells in your body, all of which use the nutrients found in the IV solution, have much greater access to them through the IV than they would through food. The IV produces a much higher concentration of nutrients in the bloodstream. It "fills in the cracks" lost to everyday depletions as well as to more significant causes of depletion (such as injury) that normal digestion cannot address.
>
> Of course, this does not mean that, if you get the IV, you don't need to eat well or that you can eat whatever you want. A healthy diet is also essential to good health—though it, too, is insufficient alone. IV therapy *complements* nutrition by going beyond the limitations that a healthy diet runs up against.

Why IV?

When we eat, it is with the aim of getting the beneficial ingredients of the food into our bloodstream. Unfortunately, our digestion can only process so much of this material. It also has processes in place for filtering out the bad stuff, and for anything it's not going to use to be excreted—so a lot of the good nutrients in food don't end up making it all the way to the bloodstream.

Normally, nutrients taken orally enter the cell through *active transport*. This process requires cell energy and the cell's ability to transport the nutrients from outside the cell into the cell. Diseased cells lack the energy and the ability required to absorb nutrients effectively, thus decreasing the amount of nutrients that reach the cell.

With IV therapy, nutrients enter the cell without using the cell's active transport. They can be used by our cells and transported to our organs, joints, ligaments, and other key destinations in the body right away.

With trillions of cells in your body, and limited access to micronutrients, the demand ends up being much greater than the supply—which is what leads cells and various pathways to break down or not function as well, thus leading to a wide variety of potential health problems. The IV provides that supply—it floods the market, in a sense, so that the hungry cells have much greater access to the nutrients that nourish them. In fact, IV therapy can result in concentrations of micronutrients in the blood that are higher than is even possible to obtain through oral intake alone.

In some cases, IV therapy is actually *healthier* than eating as a way to replenish certain nutrients.

For instance, a normal daily dose of oral vitamin C is 1000-3000 mg (in divided doses), only a portion of which actually reaches the bloodstream. If you take a higher dose of vitamin C orally in an effort to get even more vitamin C, you will likely have very loose stools or diarrhea, and your kidneys will filter out the excess. Alternatively, through IV administration, doses up to 100 grams can be achieved, all at once, without the digestive side effects from oral intake. (You couldn't possibly ingest 100g of vitamin C orally!)

These changes at the micro level have macro consequences. Your health is determined by the health of the cells that make up your body. Each cell requires a combination of vitamins, minerals, amino acids, lipids, and hydration for the thousands of biochemical reactions performed every second of every day. Chronic deficiency of any one of these nutrients is the most frequent cause of cellular dysfunction, cellular aging, and the manifestation of symptoms and disease.

Deficiencies are typically not medical emergencies, which is why we can easily overlook them. Some (functional deficiencies) may not even manifest clearly (we function just fine). *True* (as opposed to functional) deficiencies lead to specific symptoms occurring very clearly. If you are experiencing hair loss, brittle nails, poor iron absorption, dry skin, cracked skin, nerve tingling, numbness, muscle cramps, changes in stool, low energy, or migraines (to name a few), you are likely experiencing the result of a nutrient deficiency. You don't have to live this way; this can be fixed!

If you're wondering how we can know if we have functional deficiencies if no symptoms manifest, there is testing that looks at how well the body utilizes vitamins, minerals, amino/fatty acids, antioxidants, and metabolites, while conveying the body's need for these micronutrients that enable the body to produce enzymes, hormones, and other substances essential for proper growth, development, and good health.[42]

Advances in research and technology allow us to study how nutrients function within our cells, and we can appreciate why having too little of these important nutrients can lead to low energy, early aging, and disharmony in the body—eventually leading to disease.

---

42 "NutrEval® FMV," Geneva Diagnostics, accessed September 30, 2022, https://www.gdx.net/product/nutreval-fmv-nutritional-test-blood-urine.

Equally powerful, we can help reverse chronic disease with targeted nutrient repletion. For example, low magnesium often causes constipation. Low B vitamins can cause cracks in the side of your mouth. Low B12 can cause decreased nerve ending sensation. Low vitamin D can decrease immune function and slow recovery time. Replenish the nutrient status, and these symptoms can improve.

> ## YOUR FIRST VISIT
>
> On your first visit, we take a deep dive into your medical history, family history, head-to-toe symptoms, and key areas of wellness—like digestion, stress, and sleep.
>
> My favorite question I ask is: "What's your vision for your health? When we sit down again in three months, how do you want to feel?"
>
> Together, we build a context for your vision of wellness and establish how to get you there. We review your nutrient intake from food to supplementation and medications, as well as how you are nourishing your mind, body, and cells. (More on this in chapter 4.)
>
> We then do a physical exam, which includes an assessment of blood pressure, pulse oxygenation, heart rate, and other clinically relevant physical assessments. We look at your most recent bloodwork, as well as assessing if anything has been missed—for example, I often find a new patient is low in vitamin D, which hadn't been included in previous routine testing.

> Alongside your testing, we discuss the importance of micronutrients, which I share throughout this book.
>
> We examine your bloodwork before and sometimes *after* your first IV, because the first few IVs are *foundation* solutions that help prime your body to receive the customized doses we give later. Bloodwork will always factor into your care, analysis, and customization.

What's in the Bag?

The foundation IV contains a solution of small doses of the key micronutrients: vitamin C, B vitamins, B 12, calcium, magnesium, trace minerals, and the hydrating fluids saline and/or sterile water.

For instance, to match your blood osmolarity, I'll use sterile water for higher doses of vitamin C, and saline for lower doses of vitamin C.

The nutrients the foundation IV delivers into your bloodstream are the very same ones that environmental toxins and everyday wear-and-tear are constantly depleting. The foundation can thus contribute to better cellular health, and thus better digestion, brain function, energy, and more. It likewise boosts the immune system, helps your body process toxins, and can help relieve symptoms of a variety of medical conditions.

It's like you just had a super smoothie, but one where the nutrients bypass your gut and go directly into your body where needed, and at a much higher level.

IV therapy is administered as a drip, where gravity lets the IV drip down through a thin, flexible tube called a catheter into the vein. The needle doesn't stay in your vein during treatment, just the catheter tube. You can bend and move your arm during treatment since no needle remains (unless we use a butterfly needle for smaller veins, then the needle stays in).

> It's like you just had a super smoothie, but one where the nutrients bypass your gut and go directly into your body where needed, and at a much higher level.

In the foundation series of IVs, you receive 100-250 ml of solution (about the size of a smartphone case), in one bag per session. The drip lasts approximately 25-45 minutes.

After the foundation series of IVs, we often modify the mixture in various ways in order to address the needs of the specific patient. At this point, the typical IV we give is 250-300 ml, which takes 45 minutes to an hour.

Some IV therapies can be given through a push, where we use a syringe to inject the IV fluid into the vein instead of letting it drip in. This method usually takes less time to administer (5 minutes), and contains lower dosing, but is still beneficial as a boost between treatments, or when you are time-pressed. Sometimes I combine the two: you might get a drip followed by a push of an additional nutrient, or I space out the dosing (IV drip one week, IV push the next) in order to maintain momentum.

What's the Goal?

IV nutrient therapy is a systemic treatment—it impacts every system in the body.

Imagine eating an apple. You get some great nutrients from an apple; it's full of vitamin C, B vitamins, potassium, and other minerals. After the apple has been digested, some of those nutrients end up in your bloodstream. I think of this as a hallway in a school while class is in session—just a few nutrients are floating around in a mostly empty hallway.

But after you have an IV nutrient treatment, it's as if class has just let out and the hallway is crowded with students. The crowd of nutrients doesn't go back to class after a short break, however. The nutrients from an IV treatment stay in your bloodstream for about six hours. That's enough time for your cells to absorb them and put them to use.

Think of a potted plant that you forgot to water for a few days; it's looking a little droopy. If you couldn't eat right for a few days, you'd be feeling a little droopy too. Give that plant some water, however, and it perks right up, almost in front of your eyes, and stays perky for a few more days. Give yourself an IV with the right nutrients, and you'll probably feel the effects on your energy level and mental clarity very quickly—and you'll continue to feel great.

The goal is to deliver micronutrients to your cells, train your body to absorb as many as needed, and benefit from IV as part of your overall wellness lifestyle.

Is IV therapy safe?

All vitamins are water soluble. There is little chance of overdose because the doses are so low.

When people say you pee out IV vitamins, this is true. You pee out all food-based and oral-based vitamins as well. In fact, you pee out medication. Our bladders and kidneys are constantly working to clear nutrients after our cells have taken in what they need.

IV therapy is both safe and effective for just about everyone. It's been shown to be safe for both the elderly and even for kids (depending on the concern).[43]

I've given IV treatments of the Myers' cocktail to a 91-year-old on multiple medications, and it's no surprise he does really well. Why? The solution is truly *just vitamins and water,* so his body has had no negative reactions.

IV treatment is also safe for pregnant women and for women who are breastfeeding. It's safe because it's the nutrients you get naturally from your food. There aren't any drugs or foreign substances going into your bloodstream—you're just getting more of what's biologically available anyway. Because the nutrients we use are all water soluble, your cells decide what to take up and how much to let in. The nutrients don't build up in your body.

The chance of infection from the needle stick is really minimal. There's so much precaution leading up to inserting a needle into a vein. We're very careful to use sterile techniques, and it goes without saying that we never reuse needles.

On top of that, we are extremely skilled at putting the needle in. After thousands of IVs, I'd challenge anyone to find a more veteran team of vein-finders than we have on staff. Every once in a while, inserting the needle can cause a slight bruise, or there might be some

---

43 Sebastian J. Padayatty et al., "Vitamin C: Intravenous Use by Complementary and Alternative Medicine Practitioners and Adverse Effects," *PLos One* 5, no. 7 (2010): e11414, https://doi.org/10.1371/journal.pone.0011414.

slight irritation from the skin, but this can be reduced or avoided by being well-hydrated before starting the treatment to dilute the very slight acidity of the IV fluid.

But typically, the most common side effect people feel is a warming sensation. That's the B vitamins, which dilate the blood vessels, so it's a healthy sensation.

While we work with needles, and many of us have baggage when it comes to needles, our process is entirely safe, sterile, and simple.

> ## THE "IV IS FOR WHEN YOU'RE SICK, RIGHT?" ASSUMPTION
>
> I've been at fundraisers where we set up an IV pole and have someone receiving an IV. Some passerby would comment, "She's sick?!" about the person receiving the IV. The assumption is that someone who has an IV is sick. It speaks to the symptom- and sickness-model of how many of us look at our health.
>
> We have to shift to seeing our wellness as Janet does in this chapter's opening story—as an array of choices we make, from nutrition to IV. Thankfully, more people are starting to question the assumption that vitamins, vitamin therapy, and the IV are only important when you're sick.

Does IV Therapy Hurt?

A question I often get asked before someone starts IV therapy is, "Does it hurt?" Everybody has their own pain threshold, but basically, there's very, very little discomfort.

I often use a butterfly needle, which is the smallest needle possible, so most people barely feel it when it's inserted. In fact, even the most needle-phobic people are surprised at how little they feel it. Sometimes, these patients, who can't bear to watch me put the needle in, ask me when I'm going to do it. I have to tell them it's already in place! There's just that tiny initial pinch, then there's no discomfort while you're on the IV. We also have cream that we can put on that desensitizes the area.

Do you hate getting your blood drawn? Many of us are afraid of needles when they're used to draw blood. It's comforting for some clients to know that you're not losing anything by getting an IV—in fact, you're getting an extra 100-250 ml in your bloodstream! On top of that, a blood draw needle is much thicker than what we use.

You may also have a hospital or blood-drawing story where a nurse couldn't find your vein, poking your arm 15 times to get it right. I've heard plenty of those stories, and I can tell you we are vein whisperers. No vein is too difficult!

Where Do the Injected Vitamins Come From?

We receive our vitamins in vials from a licensed compounding pharmacy, which follows standardized compounding procedures to make the vitamins from a synthetic base, producing a sterile, pharmaceutical-grade end product. We also purchase sterile bags of medical-grade solution. The vitamins are pure and molecularly bio-identical to naturally occurring micronutrients.

Then at our clinic, in a sterile room designated just for compounding, our specially trained technicians, wearing sterile gowns and gloves, compound the vitamins and the solution, creating the vitamin-infused bags you see in the IV lounge.

Is It Effective?

Almost every patient I've ever given an IV to says they feel better afterward. Patients who have done a series of IVs almost always tell me how much better they feel long-term.

Such feedback is subjective, of course, but we also have objective ways of knowing whether IV therapy is effective. We can do before and after tests of urine for stress hormones. When we do the urine test again after four treatments, the results usually normalize. Not always, but it is a good marker.

Micronutrient status tests can tell us what deficiencies the patient might have; after a round of IVs, we can retest to see if the micronutrient levels rise. I usually do this testing on people who are taking medications that can deplete micronutrients. Antibiotics deplete B vitamins, calcium, magnesium, iron, and zinc. Cholesterol medications deplete CoQ10. Antidepressants deplete CoQ10 and vitamin B2. Micronutrient testing looks at the levels at the intracellular level, and multiple tests can show progress over time.

What's the IV Lounge?

We administer the IV in the IV lounge at our clinic. We walk you to a big comfy chair, put a pillow under your arm, and take your vitals: blood pressure, oxygen, heart rate. We put a tourniquet on your arm, use an alcohol swab to wipe the area, then insert the catheter into a vein in your upper forearm or inner elbow. We then connect the IV to the catheter. All the supplies we use are sterile and new. Finally, we turn on the drip in the bag.

During your treatment session, which is typically thirty minutes to an hour, your hands are free. You eat, drink, hold a book or a phone, and even use the washroom—the bag hangs from a pole on rollers that can be pushed as you walk.

Some choose to tune out and listen to their own music, while others come together and talk the whole time. Meanwhile, you're monitored and helped by our lab technicians. We have a lounge of chairs on two floors, and additional private rooms if preferred.

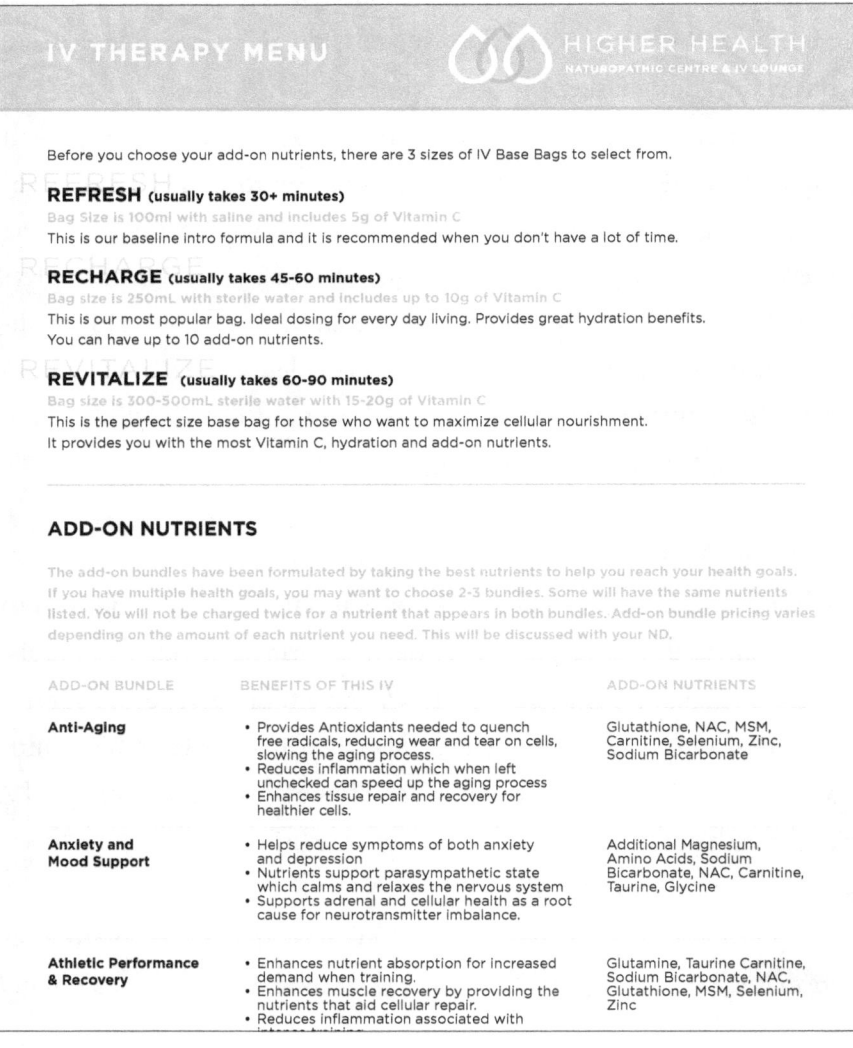

IV THERAPY MENU — HIGHER HEALTH
NATUROPATHIC CENTRE & IV LOUNGE

Before you choose your add-on nutrients, there are 3 sizes of IV Base Bags to select from.

REFRESH (usually takes 30+ minutes)
Bag Size is 100ml with saline and includes 5g of Vitamin C
This is our baseline intro formula and it is recommended when you don't have a lot of time.

RECHARGE (usually takes 45-60 minutes)
Bag size is 250mL with sterile water and includes up to 10g of Vitamin C
This is our most popular bag. Ideal dosing for every day living. Provides great hydration benefits. You can have up to 10 add-on nutrients.

REVITALIZE (usually takes 60-90 minutes)
Bag size is 300-500mL sterile water with 15-20g of Vitamin C
This is the perfect size base bag for those who want to maximize cellular nourishment. It provides you with the most Vitamin C, hydration and add-on nutrients.

ADD-ON NUTRIENTS

The add-on bundles have been formulated by taking the best nutrients to help you reach your health goals. If you have multiple health goals, you may want to choose 2-3 bundles. Some will have the same nutrients listed. You will not be charged twice for a nutrient that appears in both bundles. Add-on bundle pricing varies depending on the amount of each nutrient you need. This will be discussed with your ND.

ADD-ON BUNDLE	BENEFITS OF THIS IV	ADD-ON NUTRIENTS
Anti-Aging	• Provides Antioxidants needed to quench free radicals, reducing wear and tear on cells, slowing the aging process. • Reduces inflammation which when left unchecked can speed up the aging process • Enhances tissue repair and recovery for healthier cells.	Glutathione, NAC, MSM, Carnitine, Selenium, Zinc, Sodium Bicarbonate
Anxiety and Mood Support	• Helps reduce symptoms of both anxiety and depression • Nutrients support parasympathetic state which calms and relaxes the nervous system • Supports adrenal and cellular health as a root cause for neurotransmitter imbalance.	Additional Magnesium, Amino Acids, Sodium Bicarbonate, NAC, Carnitine, Taurine, Glycine
Athletic Performance & Recovery	• Enhances nutrient absorption for increased demand when training. • Enhances muscle recovery by providing the nutrients that aid cellular repair. • Reduces inflammation associated with	Glutamine, Taurine Carnitine, Sodium Bicarbonate, NAC, Glutathione, MSM, Selenium, Zinc

> **WHAT IF I HAVE AN ISSUE LIKE KIDNEY STONES?**
>
> You do have to go cautiously with kidney health if someone's not filtering properly, to avoid stressing their system. But the amount of solution we're giving is not actually a large volume in comparison to your whole body—it's just 100-250 ml. This amount is *not* a huge stress on the kidneys.
>
> That said, we always check kidney clearance and kidney function to know how cautiously we have to go, making their drip slower if we need to. We follow board certification guidance on all drip speeds and the amount of nutrients in every bag.

Our Specialty Training

I think it's comforting to know the depth of training our clinic has as a whole. To be a naturopathic doctor, you have to follow your undergrad with naturopathic training, graduate from a specialized IV therapy certification program, and pass a pharmacology board exam.

Per the Canadian College of Naturopathic Medicine:

> "The IVIT Certification Course is a classroom and practical course designed to ensure that Naturopathic Doctors (NDs) have the competency to both safely and effectively administer a substance from Table 2 of the Naturopathy Act Ontario Regulation (168/15) by injection. NDs will receive training to create unique solutions for injection, and prepare such products which require sterile compounding with the knowledge, skill and judgment and facilities necessary to ensure that the products are prepared

in a non-contaminated environment, free of particulate matter."[44]

On top of our naturopathic medical training, we have compounding-trained technicians and phlebotomists. Our staff has treated thousands of patients with the IV!

---

[44] "Upcoming Courses," Canadian College of Naturopathic Medicine, accessed September 30, 2022, https://ccnm.edu/alumni/continuing-education/intravenous-infusion-therapy-ivit-certification-course-2022.

CHAPTER 4

WHAT'S YOUR VISION OF WELLNESS?

When Phil looked at himself in the mirror, he saw an overweight man, in his mid-fifties, who struggled with high blood pressure, low energy, smoking, drinking, and eating. He took cholesterol medication, had joint issues, and snored nightly, not getting enough oxygen in his sleep. He wondered: *Will I make it to 65, let alone 80?*

"Quite frankly, I'm feeling a bit scared about my health," Phil said to me at the clinic during his first visit. He worried that if he didn't take care of himself now, his health would continue to get worse and worse.

Phil had recently made the healthy decision to quit smoking, but as soon as he stopped, he started gaining weight. He transferred his smoking habit to other habits like eating and drinking, which is common.

"I never felt unhealthy until recently," he said. "I never carried extra weight. I was always very active, keeping up with my kids and their busy schedules: son's hockey and daughter's dance. I set up my own construction business and run it with a team of forty under me.

The building environment is risky for workers, so it's an overwhelming responsibility every day."

As the weight piled on, Phil became more and more concerned about his overall health. It was starting to affect his daily life. "I'm not as active as I used to be. I don't have the energy to do what I want to do. Even traveling is becoming difficult—you almost have to be fit to travel and enjoy your trip. I struggle in everyday activities. It's becoming progressively worse."

Then, two people close to Phil and around his age had health scares. "My brother-in-law had a massive heart attack in his sleep. Then my best friend, who was my walking buddy, had a heart attack while walking on the day I wasn't with him. He literally walked home while having a heart attack, dragging himself in pain."

Phil had gone to a medical doctor for his high blood pressure, but didn't know much about naturopathic medicine or the IV treatment before walking into our clinic. Phil was referred to us by a friend who had a significant cardiovascular health history and who "hammered home the idea that now is the time to support my health."

"It's now or never," said Phil. He was ready to prioritize his wellness. "When I came in to see Dr. Tara, I felt my body needed to be re-energized and rejuvenated. It was like a car inspection—hydraulics, brakes, etc— with everything lubricated and working properly. I felt I was doing a proper maintenance check, from blood pressure to energy. When Dr. Tara explained IV to me, it made sense. I thought it was a good way to achieve health and healing, and faster because it was more direct."

As with every new patient, I discussed with Phil his wellness goals. "What's your vision of wellness? What does it look like for you?"

Our goal is to help you clarify how you'll feel when healthy, and how we can get there together. Sure, we talk about nourishment and micronutrients, but equally important is your perspective of your wellness.

By the end of our first meeting, Phil was able to define his vision: slimmer, well-rested, blood pressure under control, maintaining his optimal health, running again, increased fitness level, and overall improved physical strength, joint health, and cardiovascular health, with less need for medication.

After looking at his bloodwork, we then created a wellness blueprint, which showed a step-by-step wellness path to reach his goals.

At the time of this writing, Phil has made a 180-degree turnaround in his life. He's revamped his diet. He's committed to an exercise program. He has found a champion in me and those at our clinic to keep him accountable, empower his wellness, and sustain his new lifestyle. He's not perfect, but when he does get off track, he rebounds faster because he knows the consequences.

His monthly IV nutrient therapy likewise gives his cellular health a boost. "Now I do IV on a monthly basis, to stay connected and to check levels, check benchmarks, stay on track. I don't want things getting out of whack the way they were before. I like the feeling of keeping my body balanced and nourished. I'm happy I've done something for my body."

As for his health, he says, "I'm losing weight. My blood pressure is going down. I feel I have more energy."

Most important—he's discovered that wellness is fun! He's finding ways to take care of his health, and he's excited by what wellness is doing for his lifestyle. "My family notices my increased focus and commitment to health."

After building a blueprint with Phil, he's turned his life around. Now that he's reclaimed his health, he has a vision of how he wants to maintain it.

With every patient, our goal is to help them achieve higher health (it's why our clinic is named Higher Health). To do that, we first spend time with them to define their vision of wellness. We then create their "Blueprint for Higher Health," which they work from as they reclaim their wellness lifestyle. Lastly, we'll incorporate an IV routine to lay the micronutrient foundation of their health.

"What's Your Vision of Wellness?"

Every new patient starts with a 90-minute session in which we discuss their health history, their lifestyle, and their vision of wellness.

At the start of the conversation, we ask: "What's your vision of wellness? What does health look like for you?"

A new patient typically says something like, "I want to lose weight."

My reply is typically, "Sure, but how do you want to *feel?*"

I want patients to describe who they are, in their own words, when healthiest. So, when you lose that weight, how will you feel? Make *that* your vision of health: "I am healthy, refreshed, fit, active, toned, light, confident, radiant, and sexy."

> "How do you want to *feel?*"
> I want patients to describe who they are, in their own words, when healthiest.

By placing the emphasis on health *goals in addition to* current health issues, we can understand our health isn't just about taking care of one symptom or another, but about a whole lifestyle built around feeling well.

They're able to see their health in a new light. They feel a stronger sense of ownership, more control, and have greater visibility of what their health can be when they say it out loud.

This vision of wellness also shifts the conversation from a symptoms and sickness model—discussing just their health problems—to a wellness model, where we're discussing their best version of health. Oftentimes, when someone first walks in and says, "I want to lose weight," this method of describing their vision of wellness helps them talk more about their overall health than just the desire to slim down.

Chatting for an hour about health goals can be a profound experience. Few of us ever spend much time thinking about, let alone talking about, our health in a meaningful way. Health is unfortunately something we either take for granted or focus on only when a negative issue arises. Spending an hour defining vision allows me to get to know a patient well—but it surprisingly allows a patient to get to better know themselves, too!

Here are a few recent patients' visions of wellness:

- "Two months from now, I feel lighter, energized, clear-headed, and content within."
- "Instead of planning my days around getting a bottle of wine, I plan my days around health. I have reclaimed my wellness. I am fully nourished in mind and body."

- "Instead of living for my sugar habit, I listen to my body's needs. I choose healthy nourishment. I feel more focused, clear, and free."

By listening to a patient's vision of wellness, we get a holistic picture of their life, health, and goals. It's then up to us to translate the patient's vision of higher health into a blueprint that they can take home and work from. The blueprint serves as the patient's guide as they develop new wellness priorities and habits. By personalizing their goals, patients are more likely to achieve them.

Our clinic is a safe place, where patients often share with me that they are eating or drinking too much and don't know how to stop. In response, I say they're not alone. Many of us struggle with eating, drinking, and other habits that hinder our cellular health. The good news is that we can replace negative habits with positive ones that turnaround our wellness.

Often, a new patient will say, "I'm a complicated case!" They're surprised to learn that "complicated" is normal. I see many patients with a history of health issues and struggles. Not only is this normal, but oftentimes the more complex a case, the easier the treatment.

That's because "complexity" often means one's health is noticeably derailed. Getting back on track means getting back to the basics. Daily nutrition, energy, activity—these standards can improve a host of issues. For the IV, the basic nutrients likewise help address what may seem like a wide range of issues. Your situation might seem "complex," but your wellness response doesn't need to be. Even dire situations can be remedied with the basics.

Your wellness isn't a rigid list of dos and don'ts, with diet and exercise calculated to the calorie. For instance, we *don't* customize food based on your bloodwork. Instead, our goal is to prioritize the wellness decisions that give your cellular health the best support. These wellness decisions aren't always physical.

Other questions we ask to define your vision and create a blueprint:

- What are your barriers to health right now?
- What do you feel you need to do to support your health?
- What is your most negative state of health right now?
- In 1-2 months, where do you want to be?

> ## THE THREE WORDS
>
> In describing your vision of higher health, one powerful tool is to have you describe your ideal wellness in three words or phrases.
>
> A new patient, Rob, was struggling with overeating, digestive issues, and living a balanced family life. His vision of wellness focused on three words: "centered, light, and in rhythm."
>
> With three words, you can set your intention for wellness. Simple. Easy. You can grab onto the intention whenever you need to. In your day-to-day, whenever a negative pops up, you can bring yourself back to wellness with three words. These can bring your body and mind back to you.
>
> *What three words would you use to describe your health when you're feeling your best? Energized? Sober? Balanced? Every day, pick three health intentions and let those be your guide for the day.*

Bloodwork Informs Your Blueprint

After creating your context of wellness, we also investigate bloodwork, which further guides your IV treatment and establishes a baseline that we use in customizing your blueprint.

Your bloodwork reveals insights into micronutrients, lipids, hormones, inflammation, and other cellular components in your bloodstream. Elevated inflammation markers, for instance, can mean your body has systemic inflammation. Most of us even have inflammation that doesn't actually show on blood work. Due to inflammation being a common but serious issue, it's always good to treat for inflammation in the blueprint we construct.

In particular, the body wants to be alkaline (the opposite of acidic). Acidity creates inflammation. So, while vitamin C is an acidic nutrient, it actually serves to repair cells, thereby reducing inflammation.[45] We found that a moderate amount of vitamin C can significantly treat and reduce the inflammation in hypertensive and/or diabetic adults. Bicarbonate is added to most of our bags to provide additional anti-inflammatory support.

In our blueprint, we'll target your needs. These could include such health struggles we covered in chapter 1, or others which we cover in Part II:

- Low energy
- Hormone balance
- Sleep concerns
- Stress optimization

---

[45] Mohammed S. Ellulu et al., "Effect of Vitamin C on Inflammation and Metabolic Markers in Hypertensive and/or Diabetic Obese Adults: A Randomized Controlled Trial," *Drug Design, Development and Therapy* 9 (July 2015): 3405-12, https://doi.org/10.2147/DDDT.S83144.

- Digestive health (healing from the outside in)
- Thyroid health concerns
- High cholesterol
- Weight and metabolism
- Immune health
- Asthma and allergies
- Vision
- Pain

It's also important for younger people in their thirties to identify their bloodwork's baseline. If you know your current levels of the markers in your bloodstream, then in later years you can see how much you've changed. It's helpful to have a comparison at fifty to when you were thirty.

Here are some baselines that are important to know (and will thank yourself for knowing in your fifties) by getting these markers every two years at minimum—in order of importance:

- Vitamin D
- TSH
- Ferritin: TIBC, Iron, Transferrin saturation
- B12
- Hormones: free testosterone, DHEA, LH, FSH, estradiol, progesterone, first morning cortisol
    - Note: When it comes to hormones, it's important to test them at the right time in your cycle. I.e., day 3 for FSH and estradiol; day 10 for LH; and day 19-23 for progesterone.
- CRP ESR (CRP: acute inflammation, ESR: chronic/systemic inflammation)

- Cholesterol: Triglycerides, HDL, LDL, Lipoproteins
- Fasting blood glucose, HbA1c and *fasting insulin
- CBC

How Will You Support Your Wellness?

Supporting your wellness takes a lot of learning and doing. Conditions, concerns, family history, nutrition, digestion, supplements, micronutrients—wellness can seem complicated, especially when we need to account for your whole picture of health. The support plan for your wellness must be just as all-encompassing.

I like to say, "Health is hard, but it's easy." By that I mean our health can be hard to conceptualize and maintain, but once you embrace a wellness lifestyle, it becomes easy.

That's why we created the Blueprint for Higher Health, which makes a wellness lifestyle as easy as possible. That's what we need to reclaim our health—a blueprint to keep us on track.

I have a student intern who works with me. Part of her role is reviewing patient cases and asking questions. Recently, she noticed one patient had a high concentration of liver enzymes causing inflammation. That information tells me it's caused by alcohol.

As we discussed the case, I asked: "What would you do for treatment?"

"Bring down the concentration of liver enzymes."

"Right, but what's the context? Who is this patient? What does she do for work? What's her family life? What's her main concern about her health? Does she struggle with alcoholism? Is she stressed about work? Does she use alcohol socially or otherwise?"

If this is someone who has new stressors at work, and now she's hiding alcohol consumption, then they have a set of issues that go beyond "a high concentration of liver enzymes." Discussing the issues contributing to drinking will help someone feel more empowered to reclaim their wellness.

So I said, "The biggest part of her care is going to be about having a place to say, 'I'm drinking too much.' Then I can teach her about how alcohol is affecting her body, but *not* in a way where the only wellness option is abstaining. Abstinence isn't the only 'solution.' There are other options when you look at your health from a new, wellness lens of micronutrient repair and replenishment."

I can't tell you how many visits I've had with people who share they feel they're drinking too much. They're planning their next outing around buying a bottle of wine. It could be alcohol or it could be sugar—people have different habits, but they are aware of these habits and don't know how to stop.

So I said to my intern: "We must provide a safe place for them to talk about it, to help them see how five drinks a day is affecting their liver, with toxins coming into the body and causing inflammation that is making their ferritin, CRP, and liver enzyme levels rise."

That way, she's now *taking action* to help detox and *support* her body, while further understanding the impact of how alcohol is affecting her health (contributing to wear and tear and aging), as opposed to gritting it out by just abstaining.

> She's now *taking action* to help detox and *support* her body, while further understanding the impact of how alcohol is affecting her health, as opposed to gritting it out by just abstaining.

Once I'm on the same page with a patient about their wellness—mind and body—the excitement about their wellness starts to build. Often, people want to get their spouse or family members on board. Coming in together, understanding new aspects of individual and family health, receiving a reparative micronutrient IV treatment—it's fun! We even have parents come in for a health date instead of a restaurant outing.

Supporting your wellness shouldn't be about merely abstaining from negative habits. "I'm losing weight because I'm not eating" isn't a healthy or sustainable vision of wellness.

So, instead of saying to a patient, "You shouldn't be drinking—period," we make health empowering and enjoyable. We pave a pathway that makes sense for wellness, which becomes about doing what's best for your body rather than depriving you of something. By getting to the root of the issue and offering wellness outlets, we can actually change habits.

That's why we discuss and plan for how to replace the negative with the positive. We plan a shift in mindset, a shift in nourishment. We look to get our wellness to a place where we say, «I›m vibrantly healthy because I am now fueling my body with healthy foods, hydration, and exercise that feels good! I am in a healthy rhythm and I am feeling the benefits. I understand my health, and I feel better for it!»

It's about coming at your health and your choices from a healthy mindset, prioritizing what your body and mind really wants. That's how we support our wellness in the long-term. And the greatest tool we have to support your overall wellness is your Blueprint for Higher Health.

CHAPTER 5

YOUR BLUEPRINT FOR HIGHER HEALTH

Joelle was 68-years-old and training for a half-marathon when she was diagnosed with acute lymphatic leukemia. The diagnosis shocked her. She was fit, led an active lifestyle, and was always careful to eat a healthy diet.

A mother of five, she put her life on hold to battle cancer. "A year of chemotherapy knocked the stuffing out of me," she said in an interview with me for this book.

During her fight, she could feel how her body was "crying out for health and healing." So, she joined a cancer healing center for nutrition support, practiced meditation, and started yoga. Still, energy-wise, she felt depleted. "My body was full of toxicity due to the chemo. It needed more support."

That's when Joelle was referred to me. She became one of our very first clients. Eager for micronutrients to boost her healing, Joelle was also one of the first who asked for IV nutrient therapy.

The day after her first treatment, she noticed a huge improvement in her energy. We chose specific vitamins and minerals to support her system and help detoxify the toxicity of chemo. The treatment likewise improved her mental wellness and body's overall balance. She's been with us ever since.

> ## The day after her first treatment, she noticed a huge improvement in her energy

"Whenever I feel like I'm dragging, I know it's time for a treatment. At this age and stage, you have to feed your body the best you can, and to be holistically fed—body, mind, and emotion."

Today, Joelle's cancer is in remission. She credits *all* of her wellness practices—her yoga, meditation, and running; her active social life with her family, church, and choir; her healthy diet, and her regular IV sessions—with maintaining her wellness into her 70s and beyond.

Your Blueprint for Higher Health: Mindset, Movement, and Micronutrients

I share Joelle's story because, for the past seven years, I've seen how prioritizing her mindset, movement, and micronutrients has supported her overall wellness. Despite the odds, her approach has worked out tremendously for her health.

When we create a blueprint for your health, we similarly consider more than just the vitamins we use in your IV bag, or a healthy meal plan, or what exercise gets you moving, or what vision keeps you inspired—we consider *all* of it.

That's because your wellness requires a combination of these practices.

MY PROMISE TO YOU

I promise to commit myself to your best health; to support you in reclaiming your wellness. As we work together, you will bring your self-expertise, and I will bring objective, naturopathic insight to establish your key foundations for Higher Health. I will teach you to look at your health through the wellness model, rather than the conventional sickness model. I will strive to educate, support, and inspire, so you can learn what is best for your body and make the adjustments needed to truly see a difference in your health. I want to give you new insights into what's best for you.

My goal is for you to say what a client recently told me: "For the first time, I feel excited about my health." That's amazing! I want for you to be excited about your health, to keep you confident in seeing wellness as a lifestyle—a constant evolution of different aspects of your health and life. So, I promise to help you achieve wellness that makes you excited in every part of your life. I promise to be with you every step of the way, and to help you experience excitement, optimism, and action as we move you towards your highest health.

So, after discussing with you your vision of wellness, health goals, and health issues, and performing a blood test to establish a baseline, we create a blueprint consisting of our mindset, movement, and micronutrient recommendations, specific to you. This blueprint serves as a daily tool and framework, giving structure to your wellness lifestyle.

We always address every aspect of your wellness from the three pillars of mindset, movement, and micronutrients. You must see your health holistically, as a combination of all three.

1. Mindset

Mindset starts with connecting you to the deeper meaning of *why* you're doing certain things for your health. Most of us need to attach a deeper meaning to our health to reclaim our wellness. Prioritizing your wellness isn't easy; it's your mindset that keeps you going when the going gets tough. My goal is to make wellness as easy and enjoyable as possible by first addressing your mindset and connecting to your meaning.

If your vision of health starts with "being slim," you may then dig deeper to discover "being slim" really means sustained energy, following your body's natural rhythms, balancing your routine to keep your body feeling in balance, and feeling active, fit, and able to move freely and confidently through your day.

What's the mindset I want patients to walk out the door with? If I could put it all into two words, they would be: *Choose wellness.*

I want you to feel connected, excited, conscious, and inspired about your health. With this mindset, the work (and results) will follow. You will incorporate specific movement aspects and receive the nutrients you need to reclaim your wellness. Feeling good in your body starts in your mind, when you have a mindset that chooses wellness.

To uncover a mindset for wellness, I often ask clients, "What's the worst-case scenario if you *don't* take care of your health?" I recently posed this question to a client, Rob, who was experiencing knee and joint stiffness, along with stomach pain due to an imbalanced, high-acid diet.

His worst-case scenario was that the issues would worsen to the point where he wouldn't be able to play with his two young kids. That's significant! Rob found great meaning in realizing that he needed to reclaim his wellness in order to play with his kids. "Today my mindset is I take my wellness seriously, doing multiple things for me every day, allowing me to feel healthy, confident, proactive, and flexible in mind and body." He's translating his mindset into action.

In Rob's blueprint, we started with his wellness mindset. Sitting at a desk working on a computer all day, Rob had fallen out of a wellness mindset. He agreed he needed to set aside time—even just five minutes—every day to prioritize his wellness.

Before he worked on strength or flexibility for his knee, he needed strength and flexibility for his mindset. For Rob, prioritizing work over health translated to further pain, stiffness, and rigidity. Taking five minutes to incorporate "flexibility"—whether by doing stretches in the morning, going for a walk at lunchtime, or signing up for virtual yoga—would have not just an effect on his movement but foremost on his mindset, bringing more wide-range flexibility into his body *and* mind (and work schedule).

In addition to "worst case scenario" awareness, I often expand the question to, "When you are not feeling your best, what does that look/feel like?" For Rob, it was insightful for him to connect physical pain to his existing mindset and approach to health. He was able to notice where he was being inflexible and rigid from a mindset perspective. Working on both mind and body (and cells!) is how I can best support you in actually transforming your health.

When we attach deeper meaning to our wellness goals to shift into a wellness mindset, it becomes far easier to incorporate key movement and micronutrient strategies.

2. Movement

Most patients I see know the role of "diet and exercise" in sustaining their wellness.

Movement is essential, and movement encompasses more than just exercise. For your mental wellbeing, weight, circulation, and the overall health of your body's organs and systems, movement is key—in whatever form you choose! Yoga, running, dance, resistance training, swimming, focused breathing, physical therapy, to name a few—these support healthy movement, body alignment, and tissue oxygenation. Such movement has the desired effect: to keep you healthy.

That said, many of us may think, "My one-hour walk is good enough." But be sure to stress your system, because you'll create endorphins and neurotransmitters, which literally enliven you.

On top of that, certain types of movement provide more benefit than others. In particular, *weight-bearing* exercise gives you more nutrients than non-weight bearing. Exercise utilizes vitamins, so it keeps your nutrition flowing as desired. Just as important, exercise begets more nutrient *absorption*. The more you work out, the more you need, and the more you take.

Weight-bearing exercise has the added benefit of maintaining muscle mass. As we age, we lose muscle mass. We get weaker. So, you can feel better, quickly, by increasing your muscle mass. New moms who feel tired and sluggish often say, "I've aged so much in the last year!" But once you get back into a rhythm of enlivening body movement, you can turn back the clock.

That's why movement is one of the three key pillars of each blueprint.

Rob, who had joint stiffness, weight issues, and a years-long absence from exercise, ended up working with a personal trainer twice weekly. This personal trainer focused on calisthenics and regular movements with 2-pound weights.

The movement reinforced Rob's mindset, which made him physically, mentally, and emotionally stronger and more flexible. Sometimes it takes a new mindset and a gradual approach before we're comfortable with movement again as a part of our lives.

The movement also started Rob on his journey to strengthening his knee and increasing its flexibility. On top of that, Rob described to me his newfound sense of ownership of his health.

"After thirty minutes of training hard, breaking a sweat, I think more about my body the rest of the week. When I'm hungry, I choose the healthier option because I know how hard I worked during the training. I prioritize my sleep more because I know I need my rest to recover. I'm more mindful of my wellness, where before it was an afterthought. It brings me great peace of mind to know I'm doing something positive and active about my health."

The emotional and mental effects of movement are just as important as the physical.

3. Micronutrients

I spend most of my time helping patients with micronutrients, as these are my professional area of expertise.

Getting micronutrients in food becomes even more important as we age. "Diet alone may be insufficient and tailored micronutrient supplementation based on specific age-related needs are necessary,"[46]

---

[46] Silvia Maggini, Adeline Pierre, Philip C. Calder, "Immune Function and Micronutrient Requirements Change Over the Life Course," *Nutrients* 10, no. 10 (October 2018): 1531, https://doi.org/10.3390/nu10101531.

especially the older we get. Research shows micronutrients also have innumerable positive effects on our health. Nutrients in the right foods have a huge effect on our brain health and nervous system.[47]

In each patient's blueprint, our focus is on getting as much nourishment as possible, through food, supportive supplementation, IV nutrient therapy, and red-light therapy to further enhance the cellular benefit of the IV nutrients. Throughout the rest of this chapter, let's look at the micronutrient aspects of your Higher Health Blueprint.

Micronutrient-rich food

What do you like to eat? Whatever it is, let's get you the most micronutrient-rich version of that.

How can you get the most nutrients based on what you eat? Vegetables are the most nutrient-dense food. Greens, nuts, seeds, and legumes are rich in magnesium.[48] A sweet potato is loaded with B vitamins, vitamin A, C, and manganese. The more variety of veggies and healthy choices, the more micronutrients you're getting. Think about it—a salad is like a multivitamin!

It also helps to eat earlier (not later), sit down (rather than eat on the go), actually chew your food, and enhance nutrient absorption by eating in a relaxed and parasympathetic manner as we are meant to (rest and digest!).

---

[47] J. M. Bourre, "Effects of Nutrients (in Food) on the Structure and Function of the Nervous System: Update on Dietary Requirements for Brain. Part 1: Micronutrients," *The Journal of Nutrition, Health, & Aging* 10, no. 5 (September-October 2006): 377-85, https://pubmed.ncbi.nlm.nih.gov/17066209/.

[48] Franziska Spritzler, "10 Magnesium-Rich Foods That Are Super Healthy," Healthline, Healthline Media, updated October 13, 2022, https://www.healthline.com/nutrition/10-foods-high-in-magnesium#TOC_TITLE_HDR_9.

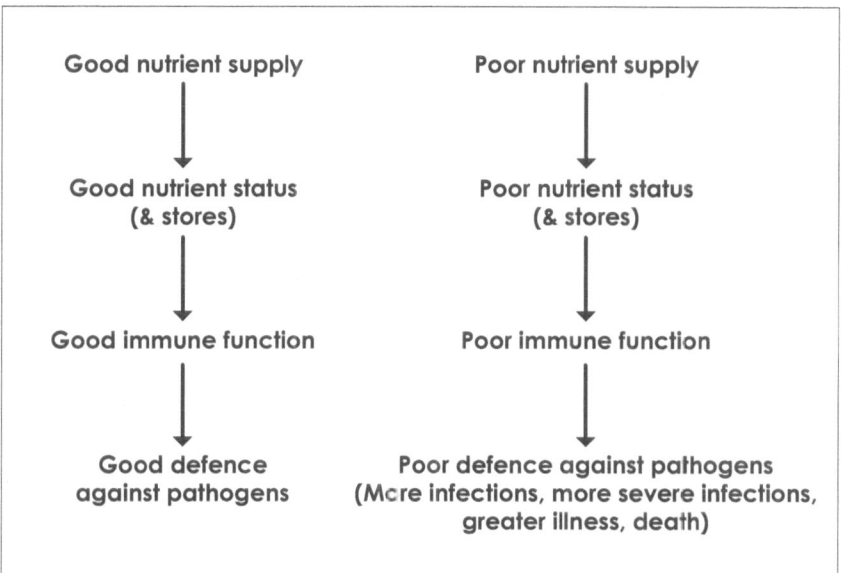

We can accomplish a lot by removing breads, pastas, and grains from most of our meals and replacing them with a healthier, more micronutrient-dense alternative. Sweet potatoes have more minerals and vitamins than a piece of bread.

If you're a meat and potato person, then have sweet potatoes instead (even better—add greens, even if that means parsley on your meal!). If toast and jam is an essential part of your routine, try avocado in place of jam or butter, or avocado with chia jam. If you usually have bread with dinner, what would be a more micronutrient-rich option? Substituting vegetables for grain can make a significant impact on your health.

Obviously, there is more to it—we've learned over time that you can't just switch your bread for salad. The point is, we *do* want to figure out how to individually increase your micronutrient stores.

What do you put in your oatmeal—sugar and milk? That's not enough. You need more micronutrients, fiber, protein, and fat. Why not chia seeds, almond butter, and blueberries? If you want ice cream or a milkshake, have a smoothie instead, and "hide" spinach or greens in the smoothie.

By loading up the food you regularly eat with micronutrients (even if you take a good-quality multivitamin with antioxidants along with your meal), you'll find you're eating a more satisfying meal. You'll notice that when you meet your micronutrient needs, you will be less hungry.

> ## When you meet your micronutrient needs, you will be less hungry.

A few years ago, I was on a vacation where I was apprehensive about the extent of and accessibility to buffet food. In order to prevent my unravelling and completely over-eating (*all you can eat chocolate eclairs? Help me!*), I chose to have the watered-down oatmeal for breakfast, rather than heavy, rich options. My rationale was that starting breakfast with a simple, non-indulgent meal may have a carryover effect to the rest of the day, creating some balance in food intake. I also took a high-quality multivitamin/antioxidant blend formula along with the watered-down oatmeal, nuts, and berries. One morning, I forgot my multivitamin, and I noticed I was *very* hungry a few hours after eating the watered down, likely nutrient-void oatmeal. People who have a set diet with more nutrients report they're not as hungry. Empty calories from sugar-rich foods keep us hungry and wanting more.

Sometimes, eating healthier is just a matter of making small changes, like making your own easy salad dressing with olive oil, lemon, Dijon, and maple syrup rather than using a store-bought dressing, which use cheaper oils that are less health-supportive and contain fewer nutritive ingredients.

It's about packing as many nutrients as you can into a meal. Overdo it on the veggies! Green vegetables, squash, sweet potato—you can fill up on these. Combine them with a moderate amount of fruit, high-fiber grains, and nuts, and you're filling your body with the micronutrients it needs.

I personally love eating a whole-food diet rich in plant-based foods, along with seasonal foods grown locally, which have more micronutrients and a higher nutrient density.

Did you ever eat a high-fat meal and crave greens, fruit, or juice afterward? Listen to your body; it'll tell you what you need. If you're feeling hungry, eat fewer empty calories and more nutrient-dense options, such as hearty homemade soups, green juices, or even micronutrient rich brownies made with hidden base ingredients like avocado, beets, sweet potato, almond flour, dates, and even spinach.

Nutrition Overview and Meal Planning

What *meals* provide micronutrient fuel and food inspiration? What recipes are tasty, healthy, and don't require a professional chef or hours in the kitchen?

Every blueprint we make also includes a personalized nutrition overview. We know how important it is to help our patients eat right. So, we make it as easy as possible with a comprehensive meal plan matching taste preferences and health goals, meeting you where you are but informing your nutrition further. We teach you how to eat for nourishment, providing you an overview of structure, inspiration, and focus for your health.

We start the meal plan with health goals, then include our recommended recipes. Each meal also shows a nutrition breakdown of calories, fat, fiber, carbs, sugar, and protein.

Even if you don't follow the meal-plan to a T, you'll know what types of food to eat, and what meal combinations to shop for. At the very least, you'll be buying a healthier selection of groceries.

Rob's Main Health Goals:
- To support healthy aging (opti-aging)
- To support joint health and reduce knee pain
- To resolve gastritis and heart burn
- To facilitate healthy weight loss
- To improve cholesterol markers
- To increase physical activity and fitness level
- To prevent cardiovascular disease (periodic arrhythmia and family history cardiovascular health)
- To support overall best health

Rob's Personalized Nutrient Recommendations
- Incorporate fundamental anti-inflammatory nutrition, which is a great starting point for joint health, digestive healing, metabolism, and cholesterol/cardiovascular support
- Within your initial consultation, we assess your current nutrition, as well as your health goals, taste preferences, time constraints, and other work/home/life factors in order to create your overview

Rob's Highlights
- Butternut squash fries with maple tahini dressing

- Celery and asparagus soup (my go-to micronutrient fuel!)
- Savory turkey and veg back (I hope your kids love this as much as mine!)
- Blueberry overnight oats
- Simple banana pancakes
- Protein-packed toast (a new spin on your current breakfast for added variety)
- Grain-free flax bread—goes well with soups and is a quick grab-and-go snack

7 days		Mon	Tue	Wed	Thu	Fri	Sat	Sun
Breakfast		Blueberry Overnight Oats	Blueberry Overnight Oats	Protein-Packed Avocado Toast	Sweet Potato & Turkey Breakfast Patties; Avocado	Simple Banana Pancakes	Bell Pepper & Spinach Egg Bake; Cucumber Slices	4 Ingredient Health Cookies
Snack 1		Make Ahead Grain-Free Flax Bread	Apples & Almonds	Hard Boiled Eggs	Hard Boiled Eggs	Apple		Green Smoothie Muffins
Lunch		Cream of Celery & Asparagus Soup; Mason Jar Lentil Salad with Tahini Dressing	Hummus & Veggie Wrap	Turkey Kale Wraps	Turkey Kale Wraps	Sesame Chickpea Mason Jar Salad		Immunity Boosting Bone Broth
Snack 2		Apples & Almonds	Hummus Dippers	Cucumber Hummus Bites	Celery with Sunflower Seed Butter	Celery with Sunflower Seed Butter		
Dinner		Coconut Turmeric Cauliflower Bowls	One Pan Chicken, Brussels Sprouts & Squash; Mixed Greens with Lemon & Olive Oil	Creamy Sun Dried Tomato Pasta; Mixed Greens with Lemon & Olive Oil	Savory Turkey & Vegetable Bake	Turmeric Chicken Nuggets; Steamed Broccoli		
Snack 3		Frozen Yogurt Bites with Berries	Frozen Yogurt Bites with Berries	Warm Apples with Cinnamon; Toasted Walnuts		Maple Tahini Dressing; Butternut Squash Fries		Tummy Soother Tea

Caption: Rob's weekly meal plan, snacks included.

	Mon		Tue		Wed		Thu		Fri		Sat		Sun	
Calories	1957	Calories	1738	Calories	2044	Calories	1329	Calories	1332	Calories	140	Calories	401
Fat	106g	Fat	102g	Fat	126g	Fat	91g	Fat	61g	Fat	8g	Fat	14g
Carbs	216g	Carbs	152g	Carbs	164g	Carbs	54g	Carbs	150g	Carbs	8g	Carbs	55g
Fiber	47g	Fiber	43g	Fiber	48g	Fiber	19g	Fiber	28g	Fiber	2g	Fiber	9g
Sugar	51g	Sugar	44g	Sugar	38g	Sugar	12g	Sugar	65g	Sugar	5g	Sugar	18g
Protein	82g	Protein	76g	Protein	90g	Protein	86g	Protein	61g	Protein	10g	Protein	14g

Caption: Nutrition facts for Rob's weekly meal plan.

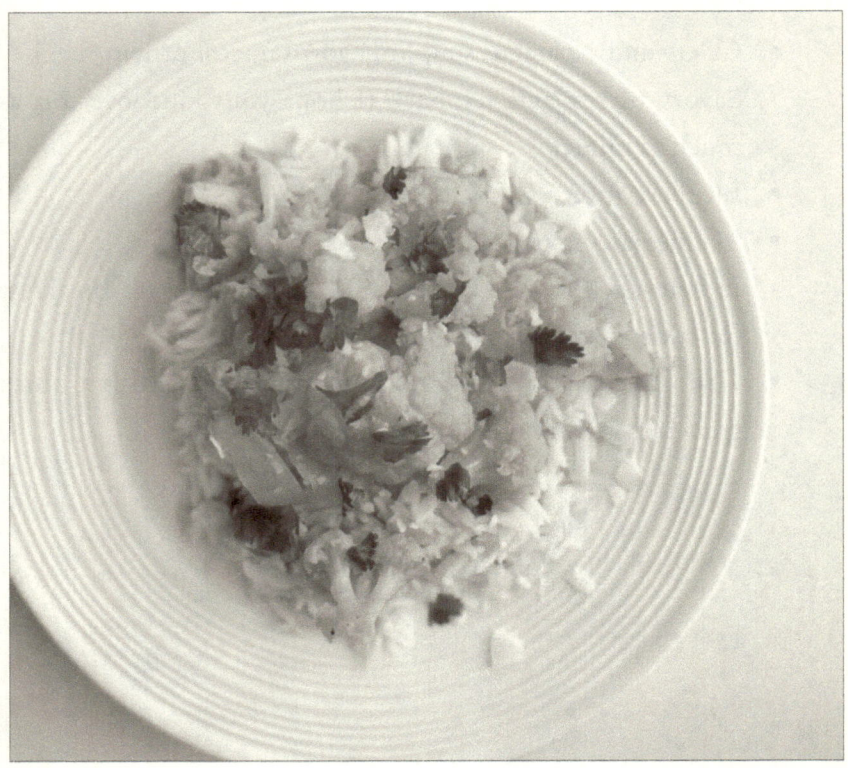

Each meal comes with a detailed recipe. Doesn't that look tasty? It's satisfying, too.

Supplements

Even with the right nutrition and IV nutrient therapy, we often need oral supplementation to provide us targeted amounts of micronutrients on a daily basis.

For Rob's stomach and joint concerns, I recommended he take a daily nutrient blend of vitamin C, Boswelia (anti-inflammatory), turmeric, collagen, MSM, glucosamine, and hyaluronic acid, which combine to serve key nourishment for cellular function, specific to joint health.

The literature on these nutrients demonstrate their use in providing continuous rebuilding of joints and tissue, including collagen synthesis (found in tendons, cartilage, ligaments and skin).[49] Exercise should be emphasized because it improves blood and lymph circulation, which enables the nutrients to reach the target tissue more effectively."

I also recommended Rob take a spoonful of apple cider vinegar during breakfast, which assists in healthy stomach acidity and nutrient absorption, minimizing gastritis, and improving cholesterol markers, blood sugar balance, and weight optimization.[50],[51]

By taking oral supplements at key times throughout the day, we can further boost the micronutrient intake our body needs.

Rob's Supplement Recommendations

- B12 sublingual, 1000-5000mcg sublingual
- Garlic (allium sativa), for immune support: 1-2 tabs/day
- Multivitamin: 1 cap/day
- Vitamin D3: 2000-5000IU/day
- Apple Cider Vinegar (ACV): 1 tbsp in small amount of water, before breakfast to improve stomach acidity and aid digestion.
- Magnesium bisglycinate, 400-80mg before bed
- Vitamin C, 500-1000mg
- B5 complex, 1 cap/day

---

49 Matthew Butawan, Rodney L. Benjamin, and Richard J. Bloomer, "Methylsulfonylmethane: Applications and Safety of a Novel Dietary Supplement," *Nutrients* 9, no. 3 (March 2017): 290, https://doi.org/10.3390/nu9030290.

50 Amir Hadi et al., "The Effect of Apple Cider Vinegar on Lipid Profiles and Glycemic Parameters: A Systematic Review and Meta-Analysis of Randomized Clinical Trials," *BMC Complementary Medicine and Therapies* 21 (2021): 179, https://doi.org/10.1186/s12906-021-03351-w.

51 Joanna Hlebowicz et al., "Effect of Apple Cider Vinegar on Delayed Gastric Emptying in Patients with Type 1 Diabetes Mellitus: A Pilot Study," *BMC Gastroenterology* 7 (December 2007): 46, https://doi.org/10.1186/1471-230X-7-46

- Glucosamine, Chondoitin, MSM (comprehensive joint formula): 2 caps, twice/day
- NAC, for antiaging, glutathione support, advanced health, immune wellness: 2 caps/day

Blueprint Labs and Tools

For each new patient, I also recommend several labs and tools so that we can best understand their wellness needs. These include:

- Bloodwork
- Subjective assessment of hormone/neurotransmitter health
- Nutrition assessment
- Additional tests

Bloodwork

When getting your bloodwork, I highly recommend you fast beforehand! We can get the best baseline of your body's functions and micronutrient levels when you have an empty stomach and there's less in your bloodstream.

In reviewing your blood, I look at a handful of important details, such as:

- Basic hematology, from red blood cells and hemoglobin to white blood cells and differential
- Cholesterol and liver enzymes, including GGT, which is an important liver enzyme and indicator of glutathione
- Inflammatory markers (ESR, CRP)
- Nutrient status: vitamin D, ferritin, magnesium, B12, vitamin C, folate

- Blood sugar (fasting blood sugar, fasting insulin, and hemoglobin A1C)
- Thyroid function testing (TSH, free T3, free T4, and thyroid antibodies)
- Specific hormone measures (LH, FSH, free testosterone, estradiol, progesterone, and DHEA)
- Kidney function and electrolytes
- Mercury exposure

Each of these markers tells me a different aspect of your lifestyle and wellness. Your lymphocytes, or your bone marrow, makes white blood cells, which include neutrophils as a type of white blood cell. If oxidative stress in our environment destructs white blood cells faster than our bone marrow is making new cells, we can see a reduced level of white blood cells and neutrophils.[52]

If I see low neutrophils, I know we could do more antioxidant support. This could involve changing your diet, or reducing alcohol consumption for a period. Even three months of no-alcohol and a new diet can dramatically transform your neutrophil levels, your response to oxidate stress, and your overall health.

My mom had low neutrophils. We put her on a botanical support, astragalus, and antioxidant support that I do for low white blood cells. It's an anti-aging botanical similar to echinacea, but more for chronic low immune system. After staying on it for than a month, she got new bloodwork, which showed her neutrophils were back up to the

---

[52] Joana Vitte et al., "Oxidative Stress Level in Circulating Neutrophils Is Linked to Neurodegenerative Diseases," *Journal of Clinical Immunology* 24, no. 6 (November 2004): 683-92, https://doi.org/10.1007/s10875-004-6243-4.

levels we like to see. The antioxidants helped support bone marrow replenishment of white blood cells by reducing oxidative destruction.

- For our Hormone/Neurotransmitter Questionnaire, check out: www.higherhealthcentre.com/hormone-neuro
- For our micronutrient assessment (Nutribody), check out: https://nutribody.ca/wordpress/nutri-body-questionnaire/

Clinically Relevant Additional Testing

In reviewing your bloodwork and discussing your lifestyle and goals, we may determine that further testing is necessary. For example, I recommend testing the current level of mercury circulating in your blood. There's a lot of mercury in seafood now. I had my mercury tested—the results *weren't* great! It's a good thing to know, especially if you love sushi or fish.

We also may recommend IgG food sensitivity testing, digestive function testing (with stool analysis), advanced hormone testing, organic acid testing, and heavy metal testing (rock on!).

Micronutrient Therapy

Of course, we can't discuss micronutrients without discussing IV nutrient therapy. I customize your IV primarily from our clinical assessment, not just bloodwork. After the first foundational sessions, which is a standard bag for everyone, we may recommend additional IV series following a treatment plan. The series includes nutrients specific to you, and an endpoint whereupon we reevaluate your progress.

A series is usually six to eight treatments. From there, many choose a regular IV for maintenance. It all depends on their response. Some people move to monthly, then feel a dip after two weeks. Many benefit from twice-monthly maintenance. During the IV series, our patients are continuing to practice the mindset, movement, and micronutrient recommendations in their blueprint.

Remember: your wellness is a combination of choices, not just one or two practices.

> ## ROB'S MICRONUTRIENT THERAPY RECOMMENDATIONS:
>
> ### Vitamin Therapy
> - Your customized formula will focus on musculoskeletal repair, anti-inflammatory support, energy, and mitochondrial health, with neurotransmitter/hormone/stress/adrenal support
> - Ingredients: 10g vitamin C + Mg, B5, B6, B complex, selenium, trace minerals. zinc, bicarb (anti-inflammatory), amino acids, taurine, carnitine, NAC, glutathione/B12
> - Recommended Frequency: Once/week for 4 weeks
> - Monitor progress/response throughout
>
> ### Red Light Therapy
> - Benefits include injury recovery, pain reduction, anti-aging, hormone balance, sleep quality, overall mitochondrial health—light's cellular nourishment as well!
> - Photobiomodulation[53]
> - Further discuss on: www.rouge.care/
> - While IV therapy delivers micronutrients to your blood stream, Red Light Therapy assists with further delivery of micronutrients from the blood stream into the cells

---

53 Cleber Ferraresi, Ying-Ying Huang, and Michael R. Hamblin, "Photobiomodulation in Human Muscle Tissue: An Advantage in Sports Performance?," *Journal of* Biophotonics 9, no. 11-12 (December 2016): 1273-99, https://doi.org/10.1002/jbio.201600176.

Your Health Homework

Of course, after discussing your health blueprint with you, we close with your Health Homework—the actions you can take immediately.

With Rob, his Health Homework was to:

- Review his Higher Health blueprint
- Prioritize the oral joint nutrients for his current health goals
- Fill out the Hormone/Neurotransmitter Questionnaire
- Fill out the diet diary/health tracker
- Start meal planning and implementing nutrition recommendations at your pace (to discuss further and monitor)

Your Wellness Tomorrow

We've covered a lot in this chapter! It's natural for any of these topics to feel overwhelming. Prioritizing your wellness can seem belabored and even awkward when we first begin. But after you start practicing, it develops into a regular part of your life.

One morning in the near future, you'll wake up and no longer think about the many components of your wellness—you'll just do them naturally. *Choose wellness* will be your mindset. You'll spend five minutes doing a mindful breathing exercise. You'll get in twenty minutes of weight-bearing movement. You'll go in for a maintenance IV therapy session. You'll cook and eat micronutrient-rich meals.

At the end of the day, wellness is as simple as repeatedly asking: *What do I need to nourish myself right now?*

Our wellness blueprint shows you several personalized strategies for you to choose wellness. With consistent effort in taking these small steps on a daily basis, health is within your control again.

PART II
Your How-To Guide to IV & Micronutrient Wellness

> "I believe that you can, by taking some simple and inexpensive measures, extend your life and your years of well-being. My most important recommendation is that you take vitamins every day in optimum amounts, to supplement the vitamins you receive in your food."
>
> — **LINUS PAULING, NOBEL PRIZE LAUREATE**

HOW IV VITAMIN THERAPY CAN HELP YOU...

1. Improve low energy
2. Support digestion (gut health)
3. Care for your vision
4. Support your immune system
5. Promote weight loss and benefit metabolism
6. Support surgery recovery
7. Reduce menstrual cramping
8. Alleviate allergies
9. Support brain health
10. Address brain fog
11. Improve Degenerctive Disc Disease
12. Support postpartum depression
13. Enhance skin health
14. Support fertility and PCOS
15. Alleviate migraines and concussion issues
16. Get better quality sleep
17. Support fibromyalgia
18. Improve cardiovascular health
19. Enhance physical performance
20. Support Opti-Aging

1. IMPROVE LOW ENERGY

The most common symptom we see on a daily basis is fatigue (low energy).

People often ask:

- Why am I feeling so tired, sluggish, and unmotivated?
- How can I improve my energy?
- Will I ever feel good and enjoy life again?

My naturopathic medicine practice changed when I first started incorporating IV therapy as part of our treatment protocol for low energy. When patients presented with low energy, I began recommending IV nutrient therapy at a frequency of once a week for four weeks, as an important part of the overall plan.

I knew the IV would improve mitochondrial function (AKA cellular energy), which in turn enhances adrenal reserves, cellular health, nutrient status, and overall body function by providing your body the baseline nutrients it needs in the most direct and therapeutic way possible—through intravenous administration.

When combined with mentorship and wellness guidance from our specialists, many clients started feeling better, faster.

Before I knew it, my "IV Lounge" was growing on referral (family members, friends, husbands/wives, and more).

The typical IV response:

- Some patients experience dramatic benefits after just one treatment, but most require a set frequency of weekly or bi-weekly treatments for four to ten weeks
- Benefits includes a feeling of lightness, more clarity, more stamina, feeling refreshed, and "like a light switch has turned on again"

IV nutrient therapy isn't complicated. It provides hydration and micro-nutrients (what your cells use on a daily basis to function), enhancing your cellular function and your body's functioning, which directly and indirectly relieves your fatigue and low energy. (For more specifics, check out: https://www.higherhealthcentre.com/low-energy/)

The nutrients:

- Vitamin C
- Magnesium
- B12
- B1, B2, B3, B5, B6
- Amino acids (full spectrum as well as additional carnitine, glutamine, glycine, taurine)
- Additional antioxidants (Selenium, NAC, Glutathione)
- Vitamin D (inserted separately since it is a fat-soluble vitamin. IV drip therapy contains water-soluble ingredients so you don't reach overdose point)
- Calcium and trace minerals

Hello, Energy! I've missed you. Welcome back!

2. SUPPORT DIGESTION (GUT HEALTH)

If you have digestive concerns, then IV therapy should be part of your wellness plan. This is especially true for:

- Inflammatory bowel disease like colitis or Crohn's
- IBS
- Celiac disease
- Leaky gut
- SIBO

Naturopathic medicine emphasizes healing from the inside out. Specific to digestive healing, IV nutrient therapy heals *from the outside in*. (Think of your bloodstream as the outer supply of nutrients, and your digestive lining as the inner supply of nutrients.)

Inward to Outward: When we eat for health, we aim to maximize nutrient density from our food choices, and then to optimize nutrient absorption from a healthy digestive lining. This, in turn, enhances the quality of our blood supply and delivers nutrients to all parts of our body. In other words, you can improve your gut health by eating nutrient rich foods—but there's a BIG CATCH. **What if you have a digestive issue where you can't eat or absorb these foods?**

Impaired Inward to Outward Healing: With most digestive health concerns, absorption is already compromised by:

- Inflammation
- Bacterial imbalances
- Immunoglobulin deficiencies
- Enzymatic deficiencies

When these issues are present, it takes longer to heal through food alone—simply because you can't absorb as many nutrients at a rate needed for health and healing. Lower absorption further delays delivery of optimal nutrition to the body, leading to overall nutrient and cellular deficiencies. Nutrient depletions then contribute to a whole host of health issues including fatigue, low energy, weakened immune function, anxiety, depression, allergies, hormone imbalances, skin concerns, and more.

Thankfully, there's hope.

Outward to Inward: IV therapy is great for people who suffer from digestive issues because it delivers nutrients directly into the bloodstream, completely bypassing the digestive tract. This ensures that our cells get the nutrients they need to function, produce energy, clear out waste, and repair damage caused by oxidative stress and inflammation.

IV therapy likewise allows the delivery of specific amino acids and other nutrients that help heal the gut. In the digestive formula,

I add sodium bicarbonate to combat inflammation as well as vitamin C and glutamine to help repair the gut lining.[54], [55]

Bottom line: *In digestive health concerns where nutrient absorption is compromised, IV nutrient therapy is a beneficial component of the care plan* by ensuring your body receives optimal nutrition for cellular health; improving antioxidant status; reducing overall body inflammation; and supporting antimicrobial benefits, repair, and replenishment.

> **CHECK OUT OUR DIGESTION BLOG!**
>
> https://www.higherheathcentre.com/digestion-iv-drip/

---

[54] Daren K. Heyland et al., "REducing Deaths Due to OXidative Stress (The REDOXS © Study): Rationale and Study Design for a Randomized Trial of Glutamine and Antioxidant Supplementation in Critically-Ill Patients," *Proceedings of the Nutrition Society* 65, no. 3 (August 2006):250-63, https://doi.org/10.1079/pns2006505.

[55] Maret G. Traber, Garry R. Buettner, and Richard S. Bruno, "The Relationship Between Vitamin C Status, the Gut-Liver Axis, and Metabolic Syndrome," *Redox Biology* 21, (February 2019): 101091, https://doi.org/10.1016/j.redox.2018.101091.

3. CARE FOR YOUR VISION

Oxidative damage hurts our bodies and overwhelms our cells, making it so we can't replenish, heal, or refresh the way our body needs.

What about the effects of oxidation on our vision?

Unfortunately, our vision is especially vulnerable to oxidative stress and cellular damage. New studies show that oxidative damage is a leading mechanism of degenerative and age-related eye diseases including AMD, cataracts, and retinitis pigmentosa.[56]

In conventional medicine, there are limited healing options for vision care. Naturopathic medicine gives us a few more options, as our vision is responsive to nutrient therapy supporting antioxidant health—making nutrients among the top most effective treatment options.

That's where IV therapy comes in. The IV provides nutrients in three important ways to support our vision in the face of degeneration:

1. **Potent antioxidants such as vitamin C, NAC, selenium, and glutathione** are used in treating ocular diseases. Administered through the IV, these can help protect our cells and tissues from oxidative stress.
2. **Antioxidant enzymes** (glutathione peroxidase, superoxide dismutase, and catalase) also help—but these require micronutrients such as selenium, zinc, manganese, and copper. We get these from IV therapy.
3. **Micronutrients in general** keep us away from the worst vision effects associated with diabetes and other chronic

---

[56] John G. Lawrenson and Laura E. Downie, "Nutrition and Eye Health," *Nutrients* 11, no. 9 (September 2019): 2123, https://doi.org/10.3390/nu11092123.

disease, as well as age-related macular disease, glaucoma, and other serious vision problems.[57]

Consider what nutrients could do for eye tissue when administered intravenously at up to 100 times the concentration of antioxidants taken orally!

At Higher Health, our IV therapy **vision protocol** is a **twice-weekly IV series for 2-4 weeks**, administered alongside our vision protocol acupuncture.

Eye nutrient checklist:
- Vitamin C to protect against oxidative damage
- Glutathione, because it's the most super antioxidant
- Magnesium to improve small blood vessel function
- B3 (niacin) to improve blood flow
- B12 and folic acid (folate) to protect the macula and optic nerve
- Selenium for a number of benefits—but especially because those with cataracts have a corresponding low level of selenium
- Zinc, which has a high concentration in the eyes
- Taurine, which has a high concentration in the retina
- L-Carnitine, from carrots!

---

[57] Maurizio Battaglia Parodi et al., "Benefits of Micronutrient Supplementation for Reducing the Risk of Wet Age-Related Macular Disease and Diabetic Retinopathy: An Update," *European Journal of Ophthalmology* 30, no. 4 (July 2020): 780-94, https://doi.org/10.1177/1120672120920537.

4. SUPPORT YOUR IMMUNE SYSTEM

Any cold, flu, or viral infection increases oxidative stress in your body, leading to cellular and tissue damage as well as local and/or systemic inflammation. These processes lower your white blood cell count and reduce your immune capacity, further leading to the need for anti-inflammatory, antibacterial, or antiviral support.

Conventional medicines often recommend treatments that can be immunosuppressive, adrenal depressive, and toxic in excess, all complicating your body's ability to recover. You may be prescribed an antibiotic you don't need, but taking it won't help you recover. Instead, it may harm the health of your gut, which contains bacteria you actually need to heal. This is why an understanding of naturopathic medicine can help supplement the role of conventional medicine in our wellness.

Immune health is proven to be supported with micronutrients that are:

- Antioxidant
- Anti-inflammatory
- Adrenal-hormone supportive
- Immune supportive

For example, the mono/Epstein Barr virus and shingles/herpes zoster virus are two specific viral infections that have demonstrated therapeutic benefit from IV vitamin C.[58]

As described earlier in the book, the administration of high-dose vitamin C (ascorbic acid or ascorbate) also provides specific benefits, and is a safe and effective adjunctive therapy for simple cold and flu infection to severe cases of respiratory viral infection.

In these cases, I recommend a 20g vitamin C base formula with 3-6 treatments in 2 weeks, providing significant symptom improvement and near resolution.

Immune nutrient checklist:

- **Vitamin C** is an essential micronutrient for humans because it's a potent antioxidant and a cofactor for regulatory genes and enzymes. Other important immune system micronutrients include:
- **Selenium**: Plays a key role in our immune function as it stimulates lymphocytes and natural killer cells. It helps to recycle other antioxidants such as glutathione and vitamin C, supporting the immune system further.
- **Magnesium**: Involved in immune health as it improves the ability of white blood cells to find and destroy pathogens. It is a great additional micronutrient to support overall immune function.
- **Zinc**: Regulates immune function. It helps control the immune system by slowing down the inflammatory process

---

58 Nina A. Mikirova and Ronald Hunninghake, "Effect of High Dose Vitamin C on Epstein-Barr Viral Infection," *Medical Science Monitor* 20 (2014): 725-32, https://doi.org/10.12659/MSM.890423.

that is activated by infections. This then helps protect our cells from damage.

- **Lysine**: An amino acid that is not only a building block for proteins, but also for immune cells. It helps reduce symptoms of viral infections and blocks the enzymes that virus cells secrete.
- **NAC**: A precursor to glutathione, meaning it plays a role in the antioxidant pathway. It supports the immune system by suppressing viral replication and reducing inflammation.
- **Glutathione**: Our master antioxidant, meaning it can balance free radicals (oxidants) in our bodies. Low glutathione can decrease natural killer cell activity, which compromises the immune system.
- **Vitamin D**: Helps regulate the immune response by supporting our white blood cells. It is great for strengthening immune function in autoimmune conditions.

5. PROMOTE WEIGHT LOSS AND BENEFIT METABOLISM

"**P**andemic weight gain." We've all heard of it—perhaps even experienced it? At our clinic, the topic has come up every day.

Any time I hear weight concerns, I always look at the patient's **cellular health and hormone metabolism**.

That's because while many people are doing all the "right" things when it comes to losing weight, there's often more to the story. Even though we watch what we eat, make an effort to exercise, and try to live a life of wellness, we may *still struggle to see results.*

When cellular health and hormones are deficient or out of balance, or when your cells and mitochondria aren't working well, it is harder to achieve results through the common practices of nutrition and exercise. It ends up becoming a frustrating cycle of forced effort, slow results, discouragement—recommitment—repeat.

A comprehensive, **nutrient-focused approach to weight loss** can make all the difference. It starts with focusing on your metabolism.

Metabolism is the process the body uses to break down food and nutrients for energy and to support different functions. What people eat, including vitamins and minerals, affects their metabolism. A faster metabolism burns calories more quickly than a slower one, making it less likely that a person will put on weight. A person's metabolism naturally slows down as they age.

When you're benefiting your metabolism, you're also healing cellular health, augmenting natural hormone balance, and improving full body nourishment.

Here are two reasons why I love IV therapy for metabolism:

- **Wellness**: When you meet your micronutrient needs *and* adopt a mindset of wellness, your hunger and overall metabolism changes. You begin to operate from wellness—knowing when and what to eat—and are more aware of what your body needs to function at its best.
- **The Collateral Effects**: I talk about cellular health for hormone balance and metabolism because at the most basic level, if your cells lack the key nourishment and cofactors they need to function optimally, this will have a ripple effect on all other areas of your body. Cellular health affects everything from organ systems to body balance to circadian rhythm (i.e., the sleep-wake cycle). These in turn affect body inflammation, oxidative stress status, cortisol production, and insulin response—all of which can decrease or increase weight.

To enhance your metabolism, a key strategy and aspect to any weight loss program is to focus on micronutrient replenishment for cellular health. Check out our online course on nutrients and weight loss! www.higherhealthcentre.com/online-course

Metabolism/weight loss nutrient checklist:
- **Carnitine**: Helps shuttle fatty acids into the cell to be used as cellular energy, meaning it helps break down fats in the body. It lowers triglycerides and LDL-cholesterol ("bad" cholesterol) while increasing HDL-cholesterol ("good" cholesterol). Carnitine helps reduce visceral adiposity, which is fat that accumulates around our organs. It also improves insulin sensitivity by increasing glucose uptake. These factors play a large role in weight loss.
- **B12**: Vitamin B12 is a cofactor in several reactions in the body. It aids in the process of metabolizing fats and proteins. Research supports an association between vitamin B12 and weight loss, as it increases our metabolism and provides us with lasting energy.
- **B6**: Vitamin B6 helps the body metabolize fats, carbohydrates, and proteins. It is needed for vitamin B12 to function properly. B6 is needed in several crucial pathways that support weight loss and detoxification.
- **Magnesium**: Helps convert energy from food and supports cellular respiration. There is research to suggest it can help regulate blood sugar and insulin sensitivity.
- **NAC**: N-acetyl-cysteine improves insulin sensitivity, meaning it helps our body use insulin more efficiently. By supporting adequate levels of glutathione, it can help increase fat breakdown. It plays a large role in our antioxidant pathway and supports detoxification in the body.
- **Bicarb**: Bicarbonate helps to neutralize acidic environments in our cells. It also helps maintain the acid-base balance that our body requires, resulting in a more proper functioning of our cells.

6. SUPPORT SURGERY RECOVERY

Even minor surgeries can take a major toll on your body, with healing taking weeks to months depending on the procedure performed.

Many of us know of the importance of immune support pre- and post-surgery, but did you know that your body requires antioxidants and vitamins for wound healing and tissue repair? For this reason, IV nutrient therapy can be an amazing adjunct to your pre- and post-surgery protocol.

Vitamin C is a precursor to collagen and enhances immunity and healing. Higher dose vitamin C (by IV) prior to a surgical intervention is strongly recommended because of the role it plays in your cellular health.[59]

For patients undergoing surgical procedures, we customize the IV formula to include higher doses of zinc to speed wound healing, amino acids for tissue repair, as well as sodium bicarbonate to reduce inflammation.

- Vitamin C, among other benefits, improves blood vessel dilation, leading to increased oxygenation to our tissues.

---

59 Ryoji Fukushima and Eriko Yamazaki, "Vitamin C Requirement in Surgical Patients," *Current Opinion in Clinical Nutrition and Metabolic Care* 13, no. 6 (November 2010): 669-76, https://pubmed.ncbi.nlm.nih.gov/20689415/.

- Zinc is necessary for producing collagen, which is required for scar formation. It also supports wound healing due to its role in cell proliferation. Amino Acids
- Glutamine helps to limit muscle loss associated with surgery, as our bodies naturally use glutamine to speed up recovery. They do this by taking glutamine from our muscle tissue, causing it to be depleted. It has shown to decrease recovery time and adverse events associated with surgical procedures.
- MSM
- Glutathione
- B vitamins

Pre-surgery, we'll do a frequency of 1-2 times/week for 2-4 weeks, stopping ten days prior to surgery. We'll resume post-surgery as soon as possible to support healing.

I've seen incredible healing from those who use the IV as part of surgery recovery!

7. REDUCE MENSTRUAL CRAMPING

If you have menstrual cramping, painful periods, PCOS, or other related hormone concerns, then IV therapy is a supportive component to your complete wellness plan. Many clients book their IV treatments specifically timed with their cycle in order to ease menstrual hormone transitions, calm muscle cramping, reduce inflammation, and support the associated symptoms of PMS such as:

- Irritability, increased tension, anxiety, fatigue, and heightened emotional responses specific to your cycle
- Abdominal bloating and water retention
- Appetite changes and food cravings
- Body aches and muscle tension
- Breast tenderness
- Acne flare-ups

When it comes to menstrual cramping, hormone imbalances, and PCOS, there are many contributing factors unique to each individual person, from physiological to psychological to social—all of which affect one's hormone balance and stress response. As naturopathic doctors, we decipher your most likely contributing factors, including a comprehensive assessment and symptom review, and we treat accordingly.

Where IV nutrient therapy comes into play is nutrient replenishment—specifically magnesium and B vitamins, as well as additional anti-inflammatory and antioxidant support.

Magnesium deficiency is one main underlying cause of menstrual cramping, as well as an aggravating factor of common PMS symptoms. Magnesium is known for its relaxing effect on muscles while controlling neuromuscular stimulation. Research reports magnesium levels (of erythrocytes and leukocytes) are lower in women with PMS. Symptoms are relieved almost immediately after the administration of IV magnesium.[60]

In our PMS/hormone support formula, we combine magnesium, B vitamins, antioxidants, amino acids, and bicarbonate.

- Magnesium relaxes the smooth muscle of the uterus and reduces inflammatory mediators causing pain
- Vitamin B6 is useful in breaking down and metabolizing estrogen in the body

I'm reminded of Debby, who came to our clinic after struggling with PCOS for six-plus years.

"My symptoms have ranged from physical ones such as cramping at various times of the month, mid-cycle spotting, long periods, to emotional ones such as mood swings and some heightened stress/anxiety," Debby said.

"Previously, I had tried seeing my GP, who recommended birth control to help with PCOS symptoms." But she wondered, "How

---

60 Nahid Fathizadeh et al., "Evaluating the Effect of Magnesium and Magnesium Plus Vitamin B6 Supplement on the Severity of Premenstrual Syndrome," Supplement, *Iranian Journal of Nursing and Midwifery Research* 15, no. S1 (December 2010): 401-05, https://www.ncbi.nlm.nih.gov/pmc/articles/PMC3208934/.

could I resolve my symptoms with a more targeted and therapeutic approach? I was getting frustrated."

Months after visiting our clinic and receiving IV treatments along with a blueprint, she noticed the IV "worked wonders."

Debby noted: "Following my IV treatments, I always feel more energized and refreshed almost instantly, as if I just woke up from a wonderful sleep. My muscles feel more relaxed (a little extra magnesium in the bag always does the trick!). This is very important for me as a Pilates instructor who is on her feet and exercising for most of the week. Also, it helps release tension in my abdomen from ovulation/period cramping. The boost of energy I feel from IV therapy usually lasts at least two weeks. I typically go once per month for approximately 3 months in a row, around ovulation, and then give a break before the next round. IV helps to balance my mood, keeps my skin glowing and refreshed, makes my eyes feel brighter, and overall assists me with any fatigue I feel post-period."

8. ALLEVIATE ALLERGIES AND ASTHMA

IV nutrient therapy can have a profound benefit on allergy symptoms such as runny nose, itchy eyes, sneezing, airway reactivity, and reduced breathing capacity. All symptoms of allergies (and asthma) stem from a complex interaction between your physiology and environmental factors. We often speak about asthma and allergies together, since both conditions involve an irritation of the respiratory tract.

The healing component of IV therapy for allergies (and asthma) stems from its benefit to antioxidant status and cellular health, as antioxidants improve cellular health.

Oxidative stress increases your inflammatory responses, which is what causes the typical symptoms of allergies. Research actually shows an association between low dietary intake of antioxidants and higher asthma and allergy prevalence. "Oxidative stress stimulates inflammatory responses that can lead to allergic disorders, such as asthma, allergic rhinitis, atopic dermatitis, and food allergies."[61]

One of the key anti-allergy ingredients in IV nutrient therapy is vitamin C, a potent antihistamine, antioxidant, and anti-inflammatory

---

[61] Hortensia Moreno-Macias and Isabelle Romieu, "Effect of Antioxidant Supplements and Nutrients on Patients with Asthma and Allergies," *The Journal of Allergy and Clinical Immunology* 133, no. 5 (May 2014): 1237-44, https://doi.org/10.1016/j.jaci.2014.03.020.

agent. As an antihistamine, vitamin C works to stabilize your mast cells (allergy cells) to decrease the release of histamines, which then reduces overall inflammation, swelling, and reactivity.

Less reactive = less symptomatic.[62]

---

[62] Moreno-Macias and Romieu, "Effect of Antioxidant Supplements."

9. SUPPORT BRAIN HEALTH

Many clients think of IV for brain support for issues like anxiety; depression; low mood; insomnia; memory deficit; or decreased focus, attention, or concentration. In fact, these may all be symptoms of neurotransmitter imbalances such as low serotonin, low GABA, low or high dopamine, or low norepinephrine.

Your whole body is made of protein. Amino acids are the building blocks to protein, and they are used in the synthesis of muscle (actin, myosin), skin and connective tissues (collagen), enzymes (digestion of food), hormones (insulin, growth hormone, thyroid hormone), and neurotransmitters.

It goes without saying that we need a constant supply of amino acids to maintain optimal brain health. The problem is that many people don't get enough amino acids despite eating abundant amounts.

> ## That we need a constant supply of amino acids to maintain optimal brain health.

Amino acids are a key ingredient within most of our IV formulas at varying doses. We can also increase the amount of amino acids within your formula as well as provide more targeted amino acids, depending on your concern. We can add carnitine for focus and energy, taurine for calming, and more.

IV amino acids may support cognitive performance and lessen stress levels by supporting a parasympathetic state which calms and relaxes your nervous system.

Amino Acids and Antioxidants = Brain Support

10. ADDRESS BRAIN FOG

Do you feel mentally drained or foggy? Do you struggle with memory and focus? Most often, brain fog results from nutrient deficiency, hormone and neurotransmitters imbalances, and/or inflammation and oxidative stress. Our brain-boosting IV formula can help support cognition, memory, and brain fog.

Here are the key brain-boosting ingredients and how they help:

- **Taurine:** Activates GABA and glycine receptors, which affects memory and mood. By binding to your brain's GABA receptors, taurine can provide a calming effect on your nervous system. It also stimulates new brain cell formation, providing the resources to replace aging, damaged brain cells.
- **Glycine:** A neurotransmitter with the ability to be both excitatory and inhibitory, meaning it can function both to stimulate brain and nervous system activity, or to quiet it. Glycine is often used to treat anxiety because it can have a calming effect on the brain.
- **Carnitine:** Shown to have positive effects on memory and overall cognitive functioning. Carnitine is an amazing energy-booster and improves feelings of mental and physical tiredness. It can increase circulation to the brain and has neuroprotective effects as well.

Who may benefit: Students and busy executives where mental demands are profound, postpartum baby-brain, cognitive burnout—basically anyone!

Here are the additional micronutrients essential to brain health:

- **Vitamin C**: A strong antioxidant that plays a large role in supporting mental performance. Low levels of vitamin C have been correlated with an impaired ability to think and remember. In addition, several studies have shown that individuals with dementia may have lower serum levels of vitamin C. Increasing intake of vitamin C has shown a protective effect on thinking and memory during aging.
- **Glutathione**: Our master antioxidant. It helps reduce oxidative stress and inflammation in the body. Research suggests that oxidative stress and inflammation near the brain, spine, and nerves (central nervous system) can increase the risk of dementia. Supporting detoxification helps reduce brain fog associated with free radicals and increases mental clarity.
- **NAC**: Working as glutathione's sidekick, n-acetyl-cysteine supports the antioxidant pathway, neutralizing free radicals that contribute to brain fog. It regulates glutamate levels in the brain, which is an important neurotransmitter involved in memory, learning, and behavior.
- **Carnitine**: Acetyl-l-carnitine can help improve memory and mitochondrial function. It has been shown to prevent age-related cognitive decline and improve aspects of learning. Carnitine supplementation improves mental functioning in older individuals experiencing memory loss.

- **Vitamin B12**: B12 deficiency has been associated with memory issues, confusion, and dementia. It is involved in the development of the brain as it maintains healthy blood cells and nerve cells. Vitamin B12 supplementation has shown to improve cognitive function in individuals who are deficient.
- **Vitamin B6**: An important cofactor in the production of several neurotransmitters that have an effect on memory and cognitive function. Research has found high doses of vitamin B6 to be beneficial for inattention associated with ADHD, demonstrating its effect on mental performance and focus.
- **Vitamin B5**: An essential vitamin for healthy brain function that has been shown to slow the progression of memory loss. It has also been shown to improve memory and support the nervous system through the production of neurotransmitters. Vitamin B5 is important for mitochondrial health, which ensures the production of ATP (energy) for our brains.
- **Magnesium**: A critical nutrient in support of brain health. It has been shown to improve both short- and long-term memory and reduce the risk of memory loss associated with advanced age. Research has found an association between magnesium deficiency and neurological disorders such as Alzheimer's.

11. IMPROVE DEGENERATIVE DISC DISEASE AND CHRONIC PAIN

I recently saw a 42-year-old mom of two young children presenting with costochondritis (inflammation of cartilage connecting ribs to sternum), nerve pain, and degenerative disc disease, as well as frequent migraines, IBS (constipation), and overall exhaustion. She struggled with her symptoms, which flared up worse and worse during the pandemic. She came to see me, looking for hope and healing through these challenges.

Degenerative disc disease is often described as feeling like a pillow between each vertebra. Swelling is caused by an inflammatory response, which can worsen with age. The swelling is due to a lack of micronutrients like vitamin C that are needed to produce collagen, which supports the vertebrae from deterioration—without which, swelling can intensify.

According to the researchers at the NIH, "Vitamin C deficiencies are a key contributing factor in the development of degenerative disk disease (DDD) in the elderly." [63]

---

63 Val H. Smith, "Vitamin C Deficiency Is an Under-Diagnosed Contributor to Degenerative Disc Disease in the Elderly," *Medical Hypotheses* 74, no. 4 (April 2010): 695-97, https://doi.org/10.1016/j.mehy.2009.10.041.

IV therapy for disc health includes:

- Vitamin C, which functions as a precursor to collagen
- Amino acids (carnitine, glutamine, taurine)
- Anti-inflammatory agents
- The benefits of hydration[64]

Our clinic has been using IV drips to relieve chronic pain for over twelve years. The nutrients used to target pain and inflammation are given at high doses to bypass the digestive tract. This gets the nutrients where you need them working ASAP.

Having an IV drip as part of your treatment plan is an important part of moving towards pain-free days and nights.

Some key benefits of the IV drip:

- Nutrients are known to significantly reduce pain and inflammation
- Helps block pain receptor pathways
- Offers a therapeutic does of nutrients to help with healing

Pain management nutrient checklist

- **Vitamin C:** A cofactor for collagen and elastin synthesis in blood vessels, tendons, ligaments, skin, and bone. It promotes wound healing and protects our cells from damage. Vitamin

---

64 Semih E. Bezci, Aditya Nandy, and Grace D. O'Connell, "Effect of Hydration on Healthy Intervertebral Disk Mechanical Stiffness," *Journal of Biomechanical Engineering* 137, no 10 (October 2015): 101007, https://doi.org/10.1115/1.4031416.

C significantly reduces inflammation, making it one of the key ingredients to consider for pain management.[65]
- **Magnesium:** Involved in our pain perception pathway, magnesium lowers pain by blocking specific receptors in the spinal cord that tell our bodies it is experiencing pain. Magnesium has shown to reduce post-operative pain.[66]
- **Bicarb:** Helpful with pain associated with inflammatory diseases, as it helps strengthen the anti-inflammatory response.
- **Glutamine:** Helps repair muscle tissue post-activity. It can decrease muscular pain by repairing muscle tissue and preventing breakdown of muscle by the body.
- **Glutathione:** Glutathione's role as a potent antioxidant encourages anti-inflammatory effects in the body. Pain is often caused by inflammation, so decreasing the inflammatory process in the body can help to reduce pain levels.

---

[65] Anita C. Carr and Cate McCall "The Role of Vitamin C in the Treatment of Pain: New Insights," *Journal of Translational Medicine* 15 (2017), https://doi.org/10.1186/s12967-017-1179-7.

[66] Hyun-Jung Shin, Hyo-Seok Na, and Sang-Hwan Do, "Magnesium and Pain," *Nutrients* 12, no. 8 (August 2020): 2184, https://doi.org/10.3390/nu12082184.

12. SUPPORT POSTPARTUM DEPRESSION

Think of IV therapy as "mommy and daddy" fuel. It is the best gift of self-care for new parents, especially if you are experiencing postpartum concerns, which are common.

Sleep deprivation, coupled with rapid hormonal changes and constant stimulation from your newborn, creates a heightened sensitivity and exhaustion of your nervous system. Many women experience changes in their mental health as a result. The good news is that IV therapy can help support mood, energy, and healing after giving birth.

Our Postpartum Recovery IV Formula helps:

- Replenish nutrient stores depleted during pregnancy and birth
- Boost energy
- Balance hormones
- Calm and energize the nervous system
- Refuel the adrenal glands
- Support the immune system for increased resiliency

The formula includes a micronutrient base containing vitamin C, B vitamins, calcium, magnesium, zinc, and selenium, as well as additional amino acids to improve energy and calm the nervous system (e.g., taurine, glycine, & carnitine).

Ideally, any IV drip targeting anxiety and mood is part of a naturopathic doctor's treatment plan that also includes possible lab tests, your preferred nutrition, supplementation, and lifestyle choices.

Unless specified, every IV drip at Higher Health starts with the following base ingredients before we add on for your specific goal:

- Vitamin C
- Magnesium
- Calcium
- Trace Minerals (chromium, copper, manganese, selenium, zinc)
- B Vitamins (B1, B2, B3, B5, B6, B12)
- Amino acids (which promote cellular repair and optimal function)

To help specifically with anxiety and mood support, an IV drip will include the following:

Postpartum nutrient checklist:
- **Vitamin C:** Can help improve mood and cognitive function. Research supports that vitamin C can help reduce symptoms of both anxiety and depression. Oxidative stress can be increased in individuals with depression, which is where the antioxidant properties of vitamin C come in to support mood.
- **Magnesium:** Helps to calm stress, relax the nervous system, and improve mood. It blocks the activity of our stimulating neurotransmitters and binds to our calming receptors, helping to relieve anxiety. Research shows that low magnesium intake is associated with a higher risk of depression.
- **B5:** Vitamin B5 facilitates the breakdown of carbohydrates, fats, and proteins as a source of fuel for our bodies. Ensuring

our bodies are nourished plays an important role in mood support and the overall health of our cells.

- **B6**: Vitamin B6 plays a large role in regulating mood. It is a necessary component of the pathways that create neurotransmitters such as serotonin, dopamine, GABA, epinephrine, and norepinephrine. Vitamin B6 increases the intracellular uptake of magnesium, leading to further calming effects.
- **Amino acids**: Several amino acids are precursors for different neurotransmitters that regulate mood, such as serotonin, dopamine, GABA, and more. By supporting our levels of amino acids, we can optimize the production and breakdown pathways of these neurotransmitters that have a large effect on mood.
- **Taurine**: Has demonstrated anti-anxiety effects by activating glycine receptors. It is a precursor to the inhibitory neurotransmitter GABA, meaning it can help promote calmness. Taurine has shown benefit in individuals with anxiety and depression.
- **Carnitine**: Shown to reduce anxiety and alleviate depression in clinical studies. It has an inhibitory effect on the HPA axis, which results in reduced cortisol levels. Cortisol is our stress hormone, and it is often elevated when experiencing anxiety or overwhelm.
- **Glycine**: Helps promote calmness by antagonizing the release of our anxiety- and panic-driven neurotransmitter, norepinephrine. Its calming effects on the brain help regulate mood and relieve anxiety. It also helps relax blood vessels, allowing blood pressure to decrease, which can be helpful in times of stress.

13. ENHANCE SKIN HEALTH

Skin food! Who doesn't want healthy, glowing skin? A healthy body radiates from the inside out, which shows on our skin. Lifestyle habits (the good and bad), and genetics "clearly" (skin pun!) influence your skin health. On the quest for radiant skin, why is IV therapy a great addition to the plan?

The truth is that the key to maintaining a healthy complexion doesn't come from a bottle, but it can come from a bag! Cleansers and lotions are topical beauty band-aids, whereas radiant, hydrated skin starts from within—and that all depends on your micronutrient supply.

I am a foodie first, and it's important to start with your plate. If you want the extra-hydrating, nutrient-rich, cellular edge, then that is where IV nutrient therapy comes in.

The goal for skin food—supportive supplementation and IV—is to get the nutrients into your bloodstream, which then circulates them to your organ systems, including your skin.

It's the directness of IV nutrient therapy—going right to the bloodstream at a more therapeutic level—that makes it a powerful and health promoting component to your wellness regime.

Such skin food is rich in collagen-building vitamin C and key antioxidant support like selenium, NAC, glutathione, and magnesium, as well as protein building blocks like glutamine, lysine, proline, and even anti-inflammatory action from bicarbonate—not to mention the hydrating sterile water base. Minerals like zinc and even vitamin D have incredible skin-healing benefits for conditions like psoriasis, wound healing, acne, and skin cancer.

Repair and replenish. Give your body, and your skin, the micronutrients for Higher Health and skin glow.

Skin glow formula:

- Treatment takes less than 1 minute and consists of a vitamin push rather than an IV drip
- Contains vitamin C, NAC, selenium, zinc, B12, glutathione, and bicarb for cellular and skin support
- Antioxidant- and nutrient-rich, supporting collagen production and reducing inflammation
- And it supports essential hydration!

Nutritional status is vital for maintaining normal functioning of the skin, so here's what's in the IV drip:

Skin nutrient checklist:

- **Vitamin C**: Skin contains high concentrations of vitamin C, which stimulates collagen synthesis and acts as an antioxidant. Research suggests that oxidative damage plays an important role in aging, including the aging of our skin. Vitamin C reverses free radical induced oxidative damage. Theoretically, IV vitamin C supplementation might improve skin health and slow the aging process of the skin. Applying vitamin C topically to the skin can help improve elasticity, making the skin look brighter and more youthful. Serums containing vitamin C can help stimulate collagen production. Studies have found that moisturizers containing vitamin C improved skin smoothness and moisture following application. Deficiencies in vitamin C lead to poor wound healing and increased subcutaneous bleeding due to fragile connective tissue.

- **B vitamins**: B vitamins have shown some benefit with skin aging, specifically with age spots and hyperpigmentation. Deficiencies in B vitamins can cause dry skin, acne, wrinkles, rashes, and fungal skin infections. Research has found that vitamin B5 can help with both acne and skin aging. Studies using B5 have demonstrated significant reductions in acne and skin inflammation.
- **Glutathione**: Helps protect the skin from damage that can cause wrinkles and has shown to improve skin elasticity. It is an important component in the regeneration of healthy skin. Glutathione can regulate skin pigmentation and reduce the skin symptoms associated with certain conditions, such as eczema and psoriasis.
- **NAC**: N-acetyl-cysteine has been studied for its use in dermatology, as it increases levels of glutathione and can assist in skin proliferation. It inhibits the production of inflammatory factors and is an important nutrient when considering skin health.
- **Biotin (vitamin B7)**: Known for its role in supporting healthy growth of hair, skin, and nails, biotin helps produce fatty acids that nourish the skin and improve the appearance of fine lines and wrinkles. Biotin maintains the mucous membranes of the skin, which helps create that skin glow. It stimulates keratin production in hair and can increase the rate of hair follicle growth.

- **Zinc**: Plays an important role in skin healing after injury. It has anti-inflammatory properties, making it a useful nutrient for inflammatory conditions such as acne, eczema, rosacea, and ulcers. Zinc can help protect the skin from UV damage by blocking the light waves.
- **Selenium**: A cofactor required to create and recycle antioxidants such as glutathione, vitamin C, and vitamin E. Increasing these antioxidants helps protect the skin from UV rays, pigmentation, and inflammation. A deficiency in selenium has been linked to a greater chance of skin cancer.

CHECK OUT OUR SKIN NUTRIENT BLOG!

https://www.higherhealthcentre.com/glutathione-iv-drip/

14. SUPPORT FERTILITY AND PCOS

IV therapy is a safe and effective method to deliver therapeutic doses of key fertility and hormone regulating nutrients such as B vitamins, calcium, magnesium, and vitamin C. With IV therapy, nutrients are administered directly into your veins, allowing for significantly higher concentrations than obtainable with oral supplementation.

Our fertility IV menu is specifically formulated for you and your fertility needs. We consider your medical history, fertility diagnosis (e.g., PCOS, endometriosis, low egg quality, poor sperm health) as well as other assessment tools and modify accordingly. Potential added nutrients include L-Carnitine, N-Acetyl-Cysteine (NAC), glutathione, and folate.

Fertility nutrient checklist:

- **Vitamin C:** Helps support the immune system during preconception. It increases iron absorption and reduces cellular damage, both of which are important aspects of fertility. Vitamin C helps increase progesterone production and can trigger ovulation in women. In men, it helps improve sperm health and motility.

- **NAC**: N-acetyl-cysteine reduces oxidative stress in the body, which is important, as oxidants can cause damage to reproductive cells. It has been shown to improve fertility in women with polycystic ovarian syndrome (PCOS) as it improves menstrual regularity and ovulation in these individuals.
- **Glutathione**: In women, glutathione helps protect the eggs from damage that can be caused by oxidative stress during folliculogenesis. Research has shown that oocytes with higher levels of glutathione produced healthier embryos. A deficiency in glutathione is associated with premature ovarian aging. In men, a glutathione deficiency can negatively affect sperm motility.[67]
- **Selenium**: Helps promote healthy follicles in the ovaries and maintains the health of follicular fluid surrounding the eggs. It can protect against miscarriages and birth defects associated with DNA damage. In males, selenium is required to produce sperm and can help improve semen quality as well as sperm motility.[68]
- **Zinc**: Plays a role in fertility as it helps regulate female hormone function, ovulation, and cell division. It is required for the body to produce mature eggs that are able to be fertilized. Zinc plays a critical role in sperm development and can help protect sperm from damage. Higher zinc levels are associated with increased sperm count and volume.

---

[67] Oyewopo Adeoye et al., "Review on the Role of Glutathione on Oxidative Stress and Infertility," *JBRA Assisted Reproduction* 22, no. 1 (January-March 2018): 61-66, https://www.ncbi.nlm.nih.gov/pmc/articles/PMC5844662/.

[68] Joanna Pieczynska and Halina Grajeta, "The Role of Selenium in Human Conception and Pregnancy," *Journal of Trace Elements in Medicine and Biology* 29 (January 2015): 31-38, https://doi.org/10.1016/j.jtemb.2014.07.003.

- **Carnitine**: Acetyl-l-carnitine is thought to help slow the aging process of the reproductive system. It has antioxidant properties and helps increase energy supply to the cells. Acetyl-l-carnitine helps with sperm maturation and motility, and protects sperm from oxidative damage.[69]
- **Taurine**: Found in the reproductive tract of women, Taurine plays a role in preimplantation as well as healthy embryo development. In males, it preserves sperm motility and sperm quality. Higher taurine concentrations are associated with higher sperm motility.[70]
- **B vitamins**: Vitamin B6 aids in hormone production by increasing levels of progesterone and strengthening the uterine lining, which supports conception. Having higher levels of vitamin B12 and folate (vitamin B9) can enhance fertility by supporting egg quality, ovulation, and implantation.[71]

CHECK OUT OUR FERTILITY NUTRIENT BLOG!

https://www.higherhealthcentre.com/fertility-iv/

---

69 Ashok Agarwal, Pallav Sengupta, and Damayanthi Durairajanayagam, "Role of L-Carnitine in Female Infertility," *Reproductive Biology and Endocrinology* 16 (2018): 5, https://doi.org/10.1186/s12958-018-0323-4.

70 F. Devreker et al., "Effect of Taurine on Human Embryo Development *in Vitro*," *Human Reproduction* 14, no. 9 (September 1999): 2350-56, https://doi.org/10.1093/humrep/14.9.2350.

71 Jorge E. Chavarro et al., "Use of Multivitamins, Intake of B Vitamins, and Risk of Ovulatory Infertility," *Fertility and Sterility* 89, no. 3 (March 2008): 668-76, https://doi.org/10.1016/j.fertnstert.2007.03.089.

15. ALLEVIATE MIGRAINES AND CONCUSSION ISSUES

For those who suffer from periodic or frequent migraines, I always ask, "What is the first treatment option you think of when you have a migraine?" The first answer is often pain and inflammation reducing medications, such as acetaminophen, NSAIDS, triptans, or aspirin.

Instead, I teach clients to think of hydration, magnesium, and B vitamins as their go-to treatment for relieving the discomfort of a migraine. Of course, IV nutrient therapy amplifies the benefits over oral hydration and nutrients.

The overall benefits of IV for migraines:

- Enhance hydration
- Replenish nutrient levels (magnesium, B vitamins, vitamins C and D)
- Reduce inflammation
- Improve blood flow
- Replenish electrolytes
- What's in the bag?
- Vitamin C
- B2 (riboflavin)
- Magnesium
- Glutathione

- **Vitamin C:** Can act as a prophylactic agent against migraines, as it has shown to reduce the risk of neuroinflammation after injury to the brain. This means it can target the inflammatory pathway to the brain that is associated with migraines.
- **Riboflavin (B2):** Vitamin B2 is effective as a prophylactic agent for migraines, meaning taking it prior to the onset of a headache or migraine can result in pain relief. This is the most researched vitamin to reduce the pain associated with migraines.
- **Magnesium:** Shown to benefit migraine symptoms in multiple studies.[72] It reduces the need for pain and nausea medications associated with headaches and migraines. The American Headache Society claims magnesium is as close as it gets to the "miracle" headache cure. It has shown results in both acute onset treatment as well as for maintenance long-term.
- **Glutathione:** Helps detoxify the body and brain by clearing toxins and oxidants, which can be associated with migraines. Its high antioxidant capacity can provide relief from headaches and migraines. Low levels of glutathione have been explored as a potential cause for migraines.

Migraines cannot be cured, but their effects can be alleviated by proper replenishment, and they can be lessened in frequency by lifestyle changes such as reducing alcohol intake, improving nutrition and sleep, and more.

---

72 Marcelo E. Bigal, Carlos A. Bordini, and Jose Geraldo Speciali, "Eficácia de Três Drogas sobre a Aura Migranosa: um Estudo Randomizado Placebo Controlado [Efficacy of Three Drugs in the Treatment of Migrainous Aura: A Randomized Placebo-Controlled Study]," *Arquivos de Neuropsiquiatria* 60, no. 2-B (June 2002): 406-09, https://pubmed.ncbi.nlm.nih.gov/12131941/.

Lastly, there's a growing body of research on the connection between vitamin D and migraines:

- Higher prevalence of vitamin D **deficiency**/insufficiency has been highlighted among migraineurs compared to controls.
- **Results:** The percentage of subjects with vitamin D deficiency and insufficiency among migraineurs and headache patients has been reported to vary between 45 and 100 percent.
- The present findings show that **supplementation** with this vitamin in a dose of 1000-4000 IU/d could reduce the frequency of attacks in migraineurs.
- **Conclusion:** It seems a high proportion of migraine patients might suffer from vitamin D deficiency/insufficiency.
- Further, the current evidence shows **vitamin D** administration might reduce the frequency of attacks in migraineurs.[73]

> **CHECK OUT OUR MIGRAINE NUTRIENT BLOG!**
>
> https://www.higherhealthcentre.com/migraine-iv-drip/

---

[73] Zeinab Ghorbani et al., "Vitamin D in Migraine Headache: A Comprehensive Review on Literature," *Neurological Sciences* 40 (December 2019): 2459-77, https://doi.org/10.1007/s10072-019-04021-z.

16. GET BETTER QUALITY SLEEP

The goal of our Sleep Aid IV drip is very simple: to help you finally get a good night's sleep!

Some of the key benefits of this IV drip:

- Helps increase serotonin levels for better sleep quality and reduces symptoms of insomnia.
- Supports the production of key neurotransmitters involved in calming the nervous system.
- Helps activate the parasympathetic nervous system, which helps with a sense of calmness and relaxation.

Sleep nutrient checklist:
- **Glycine:** Increases serotonin levels, improves sleep quality, and reduces symptoms of insomnia. It has a calming effect on the brain and nervous system, which helps the body reach deep sleep quickly.
- **Taurine:** Helps activate GABA receptors in the brain, resulting in a calming, anti-anxiety effect on the body. It is involved in creating melatonin, our sleep hormone.

- **Bicarb:** Helps to neutralize acidic environments in our cells and promotes detoxification. This can help repair cells, which is what our bodies do while we sleep.
- **Magnesium:** Mimics the action of melatonin in the body by helping to improve sleep quality. It helps activate the parasympathetic nervous system, which promotes a sense of calmness and relaxation. This is a must for any sleep aid protocol.

An IV drip used as a sleep aid is usually part of a treatment plan that also includes making the most out of your preferred nutrition, supplementation, and lifestyle choices.

> **CHECK OUT OUR SLEEP NUTRIENT BLOG!**
>
> https://www.higherhealthcentre.com/sleep-aid/

17. SUPPORT FIBROMYALGIA

Fibromyalgia and chronic fatigue syndrome may very well become one of the primary health concerns of the future. With rapid advances in technology that are speeding up many aspects of our daily living and work environments, it is not surprising that over 343,000 Canadians have been diagnosed with Chronic Fatigue Syndrome (CFS). Clearly, keeping up with the current pace of life is taxing on the body.

Unfortunately, some doctors that deny CFS and its common companion, fibromyalgia, are real. Other doctors have not yet learned how to diagnose or treat these two conditions.

> "Fibromyalgia (FM) is a syndrome that presents primarily in women and is characterized by generalized pain, muscle rigidity, poor quality of sleep, fatigue, cognitive dysfunction, anxiety, episodes of depression, overall sensitivity, and deterioration in the performance of day-to-day activities."[74]

Additionally, patients with chronic fatigue and/or fibromyalgia require much more time and attention, and our current conventional medical model does not facilitate adequate treatment for the care demands of a person struggling with these conditions.

---

74 Alejandra Guillermina Miranda-Díaz and Simón Quetzalcóatl Rodríguez-Lara, "The Role of Oxidants/Antioxidants, Mitochondrial Dysfunction, and Autophagy in Fibromyalgia," in *Discussions of Unusual Topics in Fibromyalgia* ed. William S. Wilke (London: IntechOpen, 2017), https://www.intechopen.com/chapters/57006.

Many patients with CFS and/or fibromyalgia struggle on a daily basis with family, work, and social activities. Our naturopathic doctors seek to address the main underlying causes of these debilitating symptoms in order to treat them more effectively.

We consider micronutrient deficiencies, hormone and neurotransmitter depletion, inflammation, emotional distress, trauma, environmental toxicity, and food sensitivities.[75]

In line with what we have been touching on throughout the book, IV nutrient therapy has a role to play in pain reduction, oxidative stress, inflammation, neurotransmitter and hormone imbalances, detoxification, mitochondrial health, and cellular repair.

With care and attention to all influencing factors, you will move through the healing process and realize a greater state of health.

Fibromyalgia nutrient checklist:
- Vitamin C
- Magnesium sulfate
- B vitamins
- Bicarbonate
- Glutamine
- Amino acids
- NAC
- Molybdenum, which is a co-factor for enzymes that help to detoxify copper and other heavy metals. With FS, there is also a molybdenum deficiency
- Glutathione

[75] Ather Ali et al., "Intravenous Micronutrient Therapy (Myers' Cocktail) for Fibromyalgia: A Placebo-Controlled Pilot Study," *The Journal of Alternative and Complementary Medicine* 15, no. 3 (March 2009): 247-57, https://doi.org/10.1089/acm.2008.0410.

18. IMPROVE CARDIOVASCULAR HEALTH

Before every IV, we assess vitals and note your blood pressure, oxygen saturation, and heart rate. This routine assessment is where we catch unexpected high or low blood pressure.

An ideal blood pressure range is 120/80 or 110/70 (even 100/60 can be normal for some).

When I see borderline elevated blood pressure, I think magnesium and antioxidants.

More and more research is being done about the connection between magnesium sulfate and blood pressure.[76] Researchers recently noted, "Magnesium sulfate may attenuate blood pressure by decreasing the vascular response to pressor substances."[77]

Cardiovascluar nutrient checklist:
- Magnesium sulfate
- Vitamin C[78]

76 Aysegül Bayir et al., "Magnesium Sulfate in Emergency Department Patients with Hypertension," *Biological Trace Element Research* 128, no. 1 (April 2009): 38-44, https://doi.org/10.1007/s12011-008-8256-y.

77 M.I. Lee, H.M. Todd, and A. Bowe, "The Effects of Magnesium Sulfate Infusion on Blood Pressure and Vascular Responsiveness During Pregnancy," *American Journal of Obstetrics and Gynecology* 149, no. 7 (August 1984): 705-08, https://pubmed.ncbi.nlm.nih.gov/6465220/.

78 Giana Angelo, "High Blood Pressure," Linus Pauling Institute at Oregon State University, written in May 2015 and reviewed in September 2015 by John F. Kearney, Jr., https://lpi.oregonstate.edu/mic/health-disease/high-blood-pressure.

- B2 (riboflavin)[79]
- Vitamin D (injected separate from the IV formula and similar to a B12 injection, but in adipose tissue)[80]

Cardiovascular health checklist:
- **Taurine**: Supports vascular wall tone, which helps maintain blood flow and ensure proper functioning of blood vessels. It protects the heart from reperfusion injury, where blood returns to the tissue and causes oxidative stress. Low levels of taurine are associated with cardiomyopathy, while supplementing with it induces antihypertensive effects.[81]
- **Glutathione**: Oxidative stress and inflammation escalates the progression of cardiovascular disease. Glutathione plays an important antioxidant role in the cardiovascular system by restoring cellular balance of antioxidants to oxidants, reducing inflammation and influencing vascular tone.
- **Magnesium**: A mineral that is critical for many bodily functions, including blood pressure regulation. Magnesium intake has beneficial effects on heart health and reduces pressure on the cardiovascular system. A deficiency in magnesium increases the risk of cardiovascular events, as it is required for the muscle fibers of the heart to relax. It has been

---

79 Helene McNulty, JJ Strain, and Mary Ward, "Riboflavin Lowers Blood Pressure in Hypertensive People with *MTHFR* 677TT Genotype," Supplement, *Archives of Public Health* 72, s1 (2014): K2, https://doi.org/10.1186/2049-3258-72-S1-K2.

80 R.K. Goel and Harbans Lal, "Role of Vitamin D Supplementation in Hypertension," *Indian Journal of Clinical Biochemistry* 26, no. 1 (January 2011): 88-90, https://doi.org/10.1007/s12291-010-0092-0.

81 Worku Abebe and Mahmood S. Mozaffari, "Role of Taurine in the Vasculature: An Overview of Experimental and Human Studies," *American Journal of Cardiovascular Disease* 1, no. 3 (2011): 293-311, https://www.ncbi.nlm.nih.gov/pmc/articles/PMC3253515/.

shown to reduce blood pressure in hypertensive individuals and is beneficial in those with congestive heart failure.[82]
- **NAC**: Improves circulation to and from the heart, a property which may reduce risk of heart attack. It simultaneously relieves the pressure on the artery walls and the ensuing damage caused by hypertension.

Lastly, it's important for us to focus on your wellness lifestyle. Smoking, exercise, diet, drinking—these all contribute to hypertension.

---

[82] James J. DiNicolantonio, Jing Liu, and James H. O'Keefe, "Magnesium for the Prevention and Treatment of Cardiovascular Disease," *Open Heart* 5, no. 2 (June 2018), http://dx.doi.org/10.1136/openhrt-2018-000775.

19. ENHANCE PHYSICAL PERFORMANCE

IV care is important for pre- and post-IRON MAN, marathons and distance running, sport events, or even just general stamina for your day. It can also help with post-workout recovery.

IV therapy enhances tissue repair and recovery, rehydration, and electrolyte balance, as well as overall cellular health for optimal functioning.

Physical performance nutrient checklist:
- Vitamin C
- Magnesium
- B vitamins
- Glutamine
- Amino acids
- Bicarbonate
- Carnitine
- Taurine

Research into carnitine, in particular, shows, "Carnitine has been investigated as ergogenic aid for enhancing exercise capacity in the healthy athletic population. Early research indicates its beneficial effects on acute physical performance, such as increased maximum oxygen consumption and higher power output."[83]

Physical performance checklist:

- **Vitamin C**: Enhances collagen production. Vitamin C is a precursor to collagen (i.e., you need vitamin C to make collagen). "Vitamin C reduces the adverse effects of exercise-induced reactive oxygen species, including muscle damage, immune dysfunction, and fatigue."[84]
- **Collagen:** An abundant protein in your body and a major building block for bones, skin, muscles, tendons, and ligaments. You need a continuous supply of vitamin C for replenishment of collagen.
- **MSM**: Glutathione and NAC: have been shown to provide anti-inflammatory and antioxidant effects. Strenuous resistance exercise has the potential to induce both inflammation and oxidative stress. In addition to glutathione, MSM provides the sulfur compound needed for optimal health. When we are deficient in nutritional sulfur, our bodies cannot properly manufacture and rebuild adequate amounts of healthy cells; we become susceptible to pain, injury, delayed recovery time, and other deleterious effects.[85]

---

83 Roger Fielding et al., "L-Carnitine Supplementation in Recovery After Exercise," *Nutrients* 10, no. 3 (March 2018): 349, https://doi.org/10.3390/nu10030349.

84 Andrea Braakhuis, "Effect of Vitamin C Supplements on Physical Performance," *Current Sports Medicine Reports* 11, no. 4 (July/August 2012): 180-84, https://doi.org/10.1249/JSR.0b013e31825e19cd.

85 Douglas S. Kalman et al., "Influence of Methylsulfonylmethane on Markers of Exercise Recovery and Performance in Healthy Men: A Pilot Study," *Journal of the International Society of Sports Nutrition* 9, no. 1 (2012): 46, https://doi.org/10.1186/1550-2783-9-46.

20. SUPPORT OPTI-AGING

With its powerful vitamins, minerals, and amino acids, IV nutrient therapy:

- Provides antioxidants needed to quench free radicals, reducing wear and tear on cells and slowing the aging process
- Reduces inflammation, which unchecked can speed up the aging process
- Enhances tissue repair and recovery for healthier, long-lasting cells
- Rehydrates and reduces signs of aging, such as fine lines and helps promote beautiful skin that is healthy from the inside out[86]
- Detoxification action improves the health of cells, helping to slow the process of cell aging

Anti-aging checklist:
- **Vitamin C:** Slows down age-related telomere shortening in human skin cells. It is a cofactor for elastin and collagen production in blood vessels, tendons, ligaments, and skin. Vitamin C helps reduce oxidative damage in the body, which

---

[86] Firas Al-Niaimi and Nicole Yi Zhen Chiang, "Topical Vitamin C and the Skin: Mechanisms of Action and Clinical Applications," *The Journal of Clinical and Aesthetic Dermatology* 10, no. 7 (July 2017): 14-17, https://pubmed.ncbi.nlm.nih.gov/29104718/.

plays an important role in aging. Applying it topically has been shown to improve skin elasticity and hydration.

- **Magnesium**: A deficiency in magnesium has been correlated with accelerated aging of human endothelial cells and fibroblasts (cells that help make collagen and repair the skin). Magnesium helps with cell regeneration and repair, an important component of anti-aging.[87]
- **B vitamins**: Have shown some benefit with skin aging, specifically with age spots and hyperpigmentation. Deficiencies in B vitamins can cause dry skin, acne, and wrinkles.
- **NAC**: N-acetyl-cysteine is a go-to nutrient for anti-aging, as it helps replenish glutathione levels in the body. By supporting the antioxidant pathway, it can help reduce aging at the cellular level.
- **Glutathione**: Helps reduce oxidative damage to brain cells associated with aging. Its detoxification action improves the health of cells, helping to slow the process of cell aging. Glutathione helps protect the skin from damage that can cause wrinkles and has been shown to improve skin elasticity.[88]
- **Carnitine**: Acetyl-l-carnitine has been shown to protect cells in the body from age-related degeneration. Research demonstrates its effects on the brain, where it improves memory, cognition, and mood. Carnitine supports the function of our mitochondria, which often declines throughout the aging process.

[87] M. Barbagallo and L.J. Dominguez, "Magnesium and Aging," *Current Pharmaceutical Design* 16, no. 7 (2010): 832-39, https://doi.org/10.2174/138161210790883679.

[88] Takujiro Homma and Junichi Fujii, "Application of Glutathione as Anti-Oxidative and Anti-Aging Drugs," *Current Drug Metabolism* 16, no. 7 (2015): 560-71, https://doi.org/10.2174/1389200216666151015114515.

CHECK OUT OUR OPTI-AGING BLOG!

https://www.higherhealthcentre.com/anti-aging/

A CLOSING WORD ON YOUR WELLNESS

Here you are at the end of our beginner's dive into IV nutrient therapy. I enjoyed writing this book, and I hope it has sparked some curiosity on how IV therapy can help improve your life and your well-being.

As a naturopathic doctor, I use IV therapy at my clinic as just one form of treatment. Our team of NDs each have their own focus in different areas of health, from mood and hormone health to digestive health; fertility and preconception planning; integrative cancer care; athletic performance; injury recovery and more.

As this book is being completed in 2023, our clinic is currently only allowed to work with residents of Ontario, Canada.

If you would like to learn more about IV nutrient therapy and how it can help you, or if you are interested in how naturopathic medicine can help improve your health, then please connect with us.

I've included this special link for anyone who has read my book to have a free consultation with myself or any of my associates at Higher Health Naturopathic Centre and IV Lounge.

Go to **app.outsmartemr.com/online-booking/421/DrTaraCampbell** and claim your free consultation.

Thank you for taking the time to read my book. Cheers to your Highest Health!

From the heart,
Dr. Tara

www.ingramcontent.com/pod-product-compliance
Lightning Source LLC
LaVergne TN
LVHW041712070526
838199LV00045B/1306